# SPELLING LOVE WITH AN

# X

# Spelling Love
## with an X

*A Mother, a Son, and the*
*Gene That Binds Them*

## Clare Dunsford

Beacon Press    Boston

Beacon Press
25 Beacon Street
Boston, Massachusetts 02108-2892
www.beacon.org

Beacon Press books
are published under the auspices of
the Unitarian Universalist Association of Congregations.

10 09 08 07    8 7 6 5 4 3 2 1

This book is printed on acid-free paper that meets the uncoated paper
ANSI/NISO specifications for permanence as revised in 1992.

Text design by Tag Savage
Composition by Wilsted & Taylor Publishing Services

Library of Congress Cataloging-in-Publication Data
Dunsford, Clare
Spelling love with an X : a mother, a son, and the gene that binds them /
Clare Dunsford.
       p. cm.
    ISBN: 978-0-8070-7279-0
    1. Fragile X syndrome. 2. Fragile X syndrome—Patients—Family
relationships.  I. Title.
RJ506.F73D8663 2007
618.92′8588410092—dc22
[B]                 2007013300

*For my son, J.P. Manion*

*for my family*

*and for all those who
improve the lives of children
with fragile X*

In this head the all-baffling brain,
In it and below it the makings of heroes.

—Walt Whitman,
"I Sing the Body Electric"

# Contents

# Preface

What follows is a love story. It is also an adventure story. You could even call it a mystery, a whodunit of sorts. Both tragedy and comedy, it sometimes has the weight of myth. It is my story and my family's story, but most of all—though I tell it for him—it is my son's story. He, J.P., is the hero.

The stories my son tells are surreal, illogical, often plotless. When I pointed this out about a story he had written for a school assignment (he was a month shy of eleven), including the fact that the title had nothing to do with the text, he replied blithely, "It's a folktale, dear."

But while I delight in the surreal—and live there of necessity quite often—I find myself falling into the old genres to tell this story. Its trajectory is universal. It is a story of how a curse became a blessing, how one myth gave way to another, of radical compensation, miraculous transformation, drastic revision. It is a story about making a new story when the old stories stagger and the plot lurches from A to B to X.

# PART I

## The Fragile Site

FRAGILE SITE: A term devised in 1969 by
Frederick Hecht to denote a heritable point on a
chromosome where gaps and breaks tend to occur.

—www.MedicineNet.com

My son, J.P., is sitting on his bed, his stuffed animals looking down from the shelf at its head. He is twenty, and though it's only 7:30 p.m., it's his bedtime. Suddenly he bursts out, "I don't know who I am!"

I swing around from the dresser, where I'm putting away clean laundry.

"I want the world to never end!" he cries. Knowing he now has my full attention, he says plaintively, "Who am I? I don't know. I don't understand."

I sit down on the bed next to him, my throat tight, trying to stay matter-of-fact. "Well, you're a young man whose parents love him very much. You have lots of friends. Sometimes it's hard for you to learn things, but you always try. You're not like other kids your age. You're very special."

"But who am I?" he repeats, as if I hadn't said a thing. Suddenly he's tired and gets under the covers.

"We can talk about this again if you want," I say.

"When?" he asks eagerly.

"Tomorrow night."

"That'd be sweet," he says with a grin.

A WEEK LATER, J.P. starts again. "I don't understand the world!" he declares dramatically.

"What exactly don't you understand?" I say.

"The love! The freedom! The passion! I don't understand!" He pauses. "I want the world to know just who I am!"

I am speechless. What can I tell him?

# ONE

# Anticipation

## *Once Upon a Time*

GENETIC ANTICIPATION: the occurrence of a hereditary
disease with a progressively earlier age of onset in
successive generations. In those diseases caused by
expansion of trinucleotide repeats anticipation results
from an intergenerational increase in repeat lengths.

—Robert C. King, William D. Stansfield,
and Pamela K. Mulligan, eds.,
*A Dictionary of Genetics*, 7th edition

Like the process of genetic mutation, the beginning of my story
is hard to pinpoint. Does it begin one winter afternoon in 1993
when my seven-year-old son's pediatrician called me with the results of a blood test for fragile X syndrome? Does it begin in the
earliest stirrings of anxiety when my firstborn still wasn't crawling
at eleven months? Does it begin when the pediatrician examined
our seven-month-old son and said, "There's something not quite
right here"? Does it begin when my egg merged with his father's
sperm in November 1984? Does it begin when my father's sperm
merged with my mother's egg more than fifty years ago? Or does
the story begin in a place and time untracked by human imagination, evoked by one scientist as "a slippage in the primordial
chromosome"?

Knowing the point of origin is a basic human urge. "Once upon a time" is not enough for us after the childish years. I want to tell you precisely how I came to this day, how my son came to this day. But the journey begins at a microscopic level that defies coherent narrative. We have images for it, and letters and numbers, but its essence is the garbling of a sequence, the antithesis of plot.

It took seven long years to find the right diagnosis for my son's delayed development. By that time his father, Harry, and I had seen five of the leading pediatric neurologists in the Boston area, a city known for cutting-edge medical research. In the end J.P.'s diagnosis would be read in his blood, in the X factor that everyone had missed.

AUGUST 7, 1985, a suburb of Boston. I wake up vomiting in the muggy morning air. I am nine months pregnant: swollen belly, swollen feet, moon face. I have been fending off preeclampsia through half of the pregnancy, and when my doctor hears that I have a blinding headache and nausea, he insists Harry drive me straight to the hospital.

For the next twenty-four hours the doctors monitor the protein in my urine, an indicator of whether I am still on the borderline of preeclampsia or have crossed over into its dangerous country. It is the first night I have ever spent in a hospital, and I feel as if I've handed over my identification papers to the authorities; I am the ob-gyn patient on the high-risk floor, no longer a woman with a name.

It is decided that labor should be induced. The passive voice rules the day, for I am in an HMO, where whatever doctor is on call when you are ready to deliver is "your" doctor for the length of his or her shift. Harry and I decide to call a friend of ours who is a neonatologist, as I desperately want a second opinion before submitting to the torture of the Pitocin drip. But while I am anxiously describing my medical condition to Noel on the phone, I suddenly feel the bed go wet. With a flash of recognition, I realize this is what the books mean when they say your water breaks. Harry calls for a doctor, and an examination shows that my cervix is already four centimeters dilated and labor is well under way. I am triumphant, feeling conspiratorial with the life inside me; both of us are determined to bypass as much medical intervention as we can.

My labor is fast and hard. At one point I ask the doctor how much longer it will be. "Oh, you'll have a baby in another couple of hours," she says airily. Since I am prepared to hear "in about five minutes," I immediately gulp out a request for an epidural, but by the time the nurse returns with the little cup of liquid I have to drink before the shot, it is too late for pain relief. My cervix is nearly fully dilated. The baby has trumped the doctors again.

Four and a half hours after my water breaks, John Patrick Manion slides into the world with breathtaking speed and so much urgency that the nurses yell to me to clamp my legs closed as they race me down the corridor to the OR. His second Apgar score is nine, and, although a little jaundice sets in on the second day, he is pronounced healthy.

"There's no doubt who the father of this baby is!" the nurses joke, observing J.P.'s prominent forehead, a miniature version of Harry's. In fact, as I bring my new son home from the hospital, I am miffed that there seems no trace of me in him at all.

J.P. WAS THE FIRST GRANDCHILD on both sides of the family. I was almost thirty-one when he was born and had received my Ph.D. in English from Boston University two-thirds of the way through my pregnancy. My mother tells a story of the Christmas I was six, when I raced up to the Christmas tree for the books piled underneath, bypassing the doll. It's not that I didn't play with dolls, but pretending to be a mother took second place to reading. At every significant moment in my life I've turned to books for answers, and pregnancy was no exception. I had read all the books for expectant mothers, and had my copies of Dr. Spock and a newer guide, *What to Expect When You're Expecting,* all ready for the day when the baby would arrive. Fortunately, my mother herself came to Boston from St. Louis, where both Harry's and my families lived, to help me care for my new infant as soon as I came home from the hospital.

Not only did I depend on my mother's experience to guide me through the confusion of those first days, but I also needed help physically. I came home from the hospital weak and ill from my bout with preeclampsia and other complications that had developed in what I remember even today as an otherwise healthy pregnancy. During the first four or five months I had felt a sense of well-being unlike any I'd ever had before, but in the middle of my pregnancy I developed a mysterious itching on my belly, which had me writhing at night and scratching the skin until it bled. This was later diagnosed as cholestasis, a temporary liver disease caused by the hormones of pregnancy.

I could never have managed without my mother in the first weeks of J.P.'s life. She planned to stay for a week or two but ended up staying for three, leaving my father alone in St. Louis. Living on takeout while she was gone, Dad eventually overdosed on his favorite pepper cheese from the deli and got a terrible stomachache, a comic reminder of how seriously he relied on her for sustenance.

But I was worse off than Dad. On blood pressure medication and slightly yellow from liver dysfunction, I was more exhausted than the typical new mother. My pregnancy had not been an easy one, nor was my recovery, despite the ease of the actual birth. Mom cared for J.P. for much of the day while Harry was at work in his law firm and I rested. In the evening Harry cooked delicious dinners for his hardworking mother-in-law and frail wife and mixed a Manhattan for each of us as the baby slept in his bassinet on the floor.

Only a first-time mother would keep the kind of detailed record that I did during J.P.'s first six months of life. It was my mother's idea, and I eagerly latched on to it as a way to demarcate one amorphous day from another. Each nap, each bottle, each bowel movement, each burp was set down on a yellow legal pad, accompanied by editorial comments: "messy BM!," "still sleepy after nap," "frantic for bottle." Within a couple of days the words *fretful* and *fussy* began to show up rather often on the yellow pad, and within five days Grandma used the word *colicky* to describe the new baby. J.P. soon developed a pattern: he slept days and cried all night. When my mother left we hired a college student to tend to J.P. during the night, but no sooner had we hired her than he reversed his pattern. She slept soundly on white eyelet sheets in our guest bedroom to the tune of eight dollars an hour, while all day long J.P.'s slowly improving mother rocked and held him as he screamed. But aside from this colic, which went away right on schedule at three months, our new son was a pixieish delight.

J.P. was almost seven months old when his astute pediatrician sounded the first alarm. She noticed that his eyes did not fix and follow and referred us to an ophthalmologist, who concluded that his vision was normal. But when the pediatrician saw him two and a half months later for an ear infection, she noticed again that J.P. did not make eye contact.

"See that?" she said, pointing to the way his eyes had a way of fleeting off to the side and coming back. "That's called nystagmus." It was so subtle, this little dance of the eyes, that I had not noticed it myself.

One thing I had noticed was J.P.'s acute sensitivity to light. As an infant J.P. was slow to open his eyes, which were navy blue at birth but became clear green in toddlerhood. In his baby book, under "Baby's First Day," I observed whimsically, "John Patrick was quiet and well behaved in the hospital. He was often observed hiding under his blanket to block out the noise of the other, less tranquil, babies." More likely he was blocking out the light. On his first real outing, at three weeks old, Harry and I took him in a Snugli to an ice cream store a block from our house. It was a bright, sunny day, the first of September, and he squinted fiercely the entire time we were outside. When J.P. was two months old, a friend gave him a pair of tiny sunglasses as a joke.

Now, my stomach did a flip as the doctor suggested gently, "We really need to do an emergency CT scan to rule out a brain tumor or other obstruction in his head." A few days later, I watched as my son's tiny body was strapped to a gurney and slid mechanically into a large metal capsule while I held a bottle in his mouth to keep him from moving. I was still on the safe side of panic, for I believed the pediatrician when she said the odds were very slim that the doctors would find anything abnormal in J.P.'s brain. Indeed, no tumor was found, but when Harry and I met with the pediatrician and neurologist three days later, they sat us down to give us some unsettling news about our son's CT scan. It showed, they said, that the ventricles of J.P.'s brain were mildly enlarged, with wide extracerebral spaces that suggested megalocephaly, an enlarged head. They quickly added that there was no known significance to this finding, but it was definitely abnormal.

My own brain was reeling, but I sought logic to prop myself up. "Is it possible," I asked the neurologist, "that the enlarged ventricles could represent something positive, some extra gift?" I was thinking about what Einstein's brain might have looked like.

"No," he said firmly, "it's not." Since he had admitted that he didn't know why J.P.'s brain was abnormal, and since he had probably never seen the CT scan of a genius, I reasoned, I didn't know how he could rule out the possibility that J.P. was special in a different way from what he was implying.

The neurologist's report for this visit, May 30, 1986, stated that he was "upbeat about prognosis," finding J.P. to be a "very bright youngster with some minimal gross motor slowness in development which I cannot at this time consider to be in the abnormal range." However, five months later, he sounded a more cautious note, for J.P. was now fourteen and a half months old and not yet walking. Although "friendly, sociable, and engaging," the doctor wrote, J.P. had only six or seven consonant sounds and no specific words; he was doing "a lot of high-pitched screeching." The report ended ominously: "His facial features remind me of a possible syndrome and in fact to some degree are reminiscent of Williams syndrome although clearly this is not the situation."

MEANWHILE, IN THE WORLD outside the doctors' offices, life with J.P. was exhilarating but subtly off kilter. In the first two years of his life I didn't work outside the home, leaving behind my university teaching for the luxury of immersion in motherhood. But the days were long and lonely, and J.P. was a skittish, easily overstimulated baby. I blamed myself; after all, I was high-strung and hated crowds and loud noises. Perhaps my baby was mirroring my own personality.

J.P. hit each developmental milestone in the baby books a little later than the one before. He sat at seven months, very close to average, but he did not crawl until two weeks before his first birthday, and then stood in his crib for the first time that same week. Now we were in a much grayer zone of normal. His body, even to this inexperienced mother, seemed floppy, in constant need of propping or holding, but when his muscles weren't flaccid, they were fiercely tensed. He would quiver with excitement, stiffening his legs and arms, a gesture that his father and I read as a charming excitability, but that I did not see in the children of my friends.

Most frustrating to me was that at eighteen months, my baby

spoke no words. He had a few sounds, but he didn't babble. Instead J.P. screeched a lot, high-pitched shrieks that unnerved me and sent me running to try to figure out what he needed. It didn't help that my mother had always claimed that I spoke my first word, "ee," for *egg*, at seven months. J.P. got frequent ear infections, and these, coupled with his developmental delays, led to a hearing test. The results were normal, as we had suspected they would be, since he seemed to understand all that was said to him even though he could not speak.

Increasingly anxious, in February 1987, when J.P. was eighteen months old, Harry and I returned to the same neurologist who had read the CT scan, and this time he was more definitive about the meaning of his latest test of J.P. On something called a Denver screen, he felt that J.P. was about three months behind.

"Can he say three words beyond 'Mama' and 'Dada'?"

"No."

"Does he imitate housework?"

"No."

"Can he use a spoon without spilling?"

"No."

"Does he scribble with a pencil?"

"No."

"Can he drink from a cup?"

"Yes." (Whew.)

The doctor remained intrigued by J.P.'s physiognomy—the large head, of course, which was measured by every neurologist we were to see in the years to come—but something else tugged at him. Like the nurses in the hospital, the doctor saw J.P.'s resemblance to Harry, but in this context he seemed to be reassuring himself: "His facial features in fact are very reminiscent of his father's with a very strong eyebrow, etc.," his report stated, and he concluded, "I did mention the possible consultation with a geneticist although I am somewhat on the fence post given the fa-

ther's physiognomy and do not feel strong about it at this time."
Neither Harry nor I remember any mention of a geneticist during
our session.

This neurologist, who practiced at Children's Hospital in
Boston, will now be called Doctor #1, for at this point, less than
two years into J.P.'s life, Harry and I were deeply concerned about
his development and decided to get a second opinion. Through a
colleague of Harry's who was a Boston native, we found Doctor
#2, a highly regarded pediatric neurologist at Mass. General and
a warm, motherly woman whose style was as embracing as Doctor #1's was cool.

J.P. made his own case in our first visit to the new doctor,
bursting into her office, attacking it at top speed, emptying out
my pocketbook and then going for the doctor's, grabbing items off
shelves, shrieking. Doctor #2, however, found him charming, pronounced his delays to be "mild," well within the norm for boys,
and told us that some boys didn't speak until the age of four. I was
deeply dubious, having heard one too many times the story that
Einstein didn't speak until four, but I felt reassured when she
thought to measure both my head and Harry's. Both of us were
found to have relatively large heads, thus allowing her to tender-
ize the clinical "macrocephaly" in her report on J.P. with the no-
tation "? familial." We were a family with large heads—big brains,
I liked to think.

That summer, the summer of 1987, we moved out of the Victorian house to which J.P. had been brought home at birth, with
its tiny sunroom nursery decorated with a cloth wall hanging
of a rabbit sitting on a crescent moon. Harry was on the move
professionally, his private law practice growing rapidly, and we
purchased a huge, Tara-like house in a tony Boston suburb. One
of its five bedrooms became J.P.'s room, with a "big-boy" twin
bed we bought from the previous owners. With ambition far beyond my talent, I decided to decorate the bed myself. On the

headboard I painted a jockey cap and a horse's head, and on the footboard I painted the starting gate of a racetrack. That's because Harry had begun to take J.P. to the racetrack on Saturdays. Their first trip was to Suffolk Downs in Boston, where J.P. crawled under the rail of the box in which they sat and was handed back by a horse trainer with whom Harry later bought his first horse. Soon Harry and J.P. were visiting Karl's stables at Rockingham Park in New Hampshire every weekend. J.P. loved everything about this weekly outing. He loved being with his father, of course, but he also loved the long drive in the car listening to country music, the visits to the stables, darting under the noses of the towering racehorses, and the open spaces in which to race around. Most of all, he loved the rituals of the track—the set intervals between races, the parade in the paddock, the thrilling call: "An-n-n-d, they're off!"

These Saturdays became my day of rest, a much-awaited respite from the emotional and physical chaos of life with a toddler whose every movement seemed random. J.P. did not play with toys so much as move them mindlessly around, throw them, mouth them, break them. His attention span was measured in seconds, not minutes. At two and a half, he had only ten to fifteen sound patterns (often the initial syllable of a word) with consistent meanings, and he continued to shriek at random intervals. He had a low frustration level and was easily overwhelmed.

Hoping to find some company, I joined a playgroup that an acquaintance told me about. As I sat at a backyard picnic table with the other mothers, I saw the other toddlers riding tricycles or clambering up a miniature plastic slide. J.P. sat with a sagging spine on the grass and flapped his hands. I began to face what I had been stolidly denying: my son was not normal.

Doctor #1 had recommended that I contact the Early Intervention Program, a state program that serves developmentally delayed children from infancy until age three. I attended one session of the program, held in the town next door, and returned home simply unable to accept that my little boy belonged with the children I had seen there. Many of their disabilities were visible—twisted necks or braced legs—and J.P.'s little body was intact; heck, it was perfect. Not only that, but I bridled at turning over my son to social services; the language of therapy and pathology grated on me, especially when I was invited to participate in a mothers' group that met while the children received therapies. What was I doing here? I thought, resisting out of sheer pride the fact that J.P. and I belonged with these sobbing mothers and screaming kids. This was another kind of playgroup, but one in which I felt just as out of place.

Still . . . sometime that year I looked into a preschool for children with special needs, telling myself this was just research in case we needed it. The day I visited Mainstay I took a step over a threshold that I never imagined crossing; there would be no retreating from this unfamiliar world, though I thought I was making my exit half an hour later, when I walked briskly to my car. I had walked into a classroom filled with therapeutic equipment, swings, walkers, mats on the floor, helmets, rails—necessities for those whose inner balance was awry. I almost fell down myself when I entered. A kind and empathetic woman spoke to me, but I heard her as if from behind thick glass. I barely held back my tears. That night I told Harry, and meant every word, that I would gladly trade my right arm—cut it off, God, now!—if J.P. could be made whole. He looked at me with alarm, perhaps fending off his own terror, but I have never forgotten his answer: "Don't be so ridiculous, Clare. It's not as bad as that." But it was.

Harry and I returned to Doctor #2 in April 1988, hoping she could give J.P. a firm diagnosis now that more time had passed. We needed words for what he was, who he was. As on our last visit, he restlessly circled in the doctor's small office, biting objects and even biting me on the cheek as he kissed me in his characteristic overexcitement. We asked, with some desperation, for her clinical assessment of J.P. But the doctor demurred: she did not have a label for our son, nor did she believe that a child so young could be called hyperactive, the term we had been using. Her report stated, "I think it may be premature to categorically consider him as a Special Needs child in the distant future, although he clearly has Special Needs on an immediate basis...." The capital letters of my son's nondiagnosis did not escape me.

A month before this visit, I had finally enrolled J.P. in Early Intervention; I was beginning to understand that I could not do for my son what trained speech, occupational, and physical therapists could do. I was beginning to let go of the brittle sense of who I was in the world: no longer the top student, the one with all the answers, but now the one who had a lot to learn. Each and every one of J.P.'s new therapists cited his inability to focus as a significant factor in his delay in their particular area. All of them felt he had potential to learn but that his attention deficit prevented him from doing so.

In search of a diagnosis of ADHD, we sought out yet another neurologist just two months after our visit with Doctor #2. Doctor #3, director of the Learning Disabilities Clinic at Children's Hospital, asked us new and quirky questions about our families. He seemed to find it significant that my family had some left-handed members and that, in the way of what he called the "black Irish," we tended to gray prematurely. We were now in the land of learning disabilities, a place with which I had a passing acquaintance, as one of my sisters had been said to have an LD in visual perception, though I'm not sure most of the family knew what it meant. I had already looked at the popular books on hyperactivity, such as *The Difficult Child,* and had seen J.P. on every page. But Doctor #3 believed that J.P.'s attention deficit was secondary to his language delay and did not award him the diagnosis of ADHD.

J.P. would remain Doctor #3's patient for at least four more years, and the diagnosis on the billing sheet always remained the same: "language delay with secondary attention deficit." Descriptive it was, but prognostic it was not. Meanwhile, although Harry and I wanted another child, I wasn't sure if I could manage another baby like J.P.

"Do we have an increased chance of having another child with developmental delays?" we asked Doctor #3.

"You do have double the chance of the typical couple, but since that chance is only one to two percent, your chances are still only two to four percent," he reassured us. Harry was a natural gambler and had introduced me to blackjack in Las Vegas, but even though I was the type to quit the table once I was even slightly ahead, I thought I could live with the odds the doctor had given us. I figured as soon as J.P. settled down a little, we would try to have another baby. I had never imagined having an only child.

Never quite satisfied with the nebulous diagnosis of Doctor #3, sometime in 1991 I took J.P. to yet another neurologist. Doctor #4 would only say that J.P. had the worst ADHD he had ever seen. I had brought him to this visit by myself, and in order to have a conversation with the doctor after he had examined J.P., I had to ask the office staff to watch J.P. as he moved ceaselessly around the office, grabbing items, mouthing them, shrieking. When I came to claim him, they were visibly relieved.

With this singularly unhelpful but oddly confirming judgment, we headed toward Doctor #5, a neurologist at Franciscan Children's Hospital in Boston, a kind and humane man whom friends in my new special-needs network had recommended. By this time, October 1, 1992, J.P. was seven years old and had a pile of medical records, from CT scans to school reports. Doctor #5's report was unsparing of the many deficits in my son's behavior, but it was clear-eyed and accurate: he diagnosed J.P. as having pervasive developmental disorder, known as PDD, and suggested that it might be worthwhile to test him for something called fragile X syndrome.

Fragile X was a genetic disorder, he explained, and in J.P.'s case it would have had to come from me, as it was passed on through the X chromosome. With unusual candor, the doctor noted in his report that at the mention of this new diagnosis, J.P.'s "parents were understandably taken aback." Perhaps that is why he was not more aggressive in recommending that J.P. be tested. Even as we were walking out of the doctor's office, Harry and I both dismissed this latest suggestion out of hand, although we had no reason more substantial than that our faith in doctors was rapidly dwindling and this proliferation of diagnoses seemed as out of control as our son. In any case, Doctor #5's three-page report ended by suggesting that it would be "appropriate to obtain a chromosome analysis for fragile X determination." It went on to note that "labeling in this way was primarily for the purpose of understanding the associated difficulties he has." There was no mention of the implications of such a genetic diagnosis, no hint that J.P.'s "label" might be reproduced on any future babies I might have or that it could cover the rest of my family with the heavy burden of a new identity.

# TWO

# Hairpin Turns

## *Doctors and Divorce*

Repetitive DNA sequences, interspersed
throughout the human genome, are capable
of forming a wide variety of unusual DNA
structures with simple and complex loopfolding
patterns.... The longer the repeat length the
higher is the probability of hairpin formation
by the Fragile X repeat....

—P. Catasti et al., "DNA Repeats in
the Human Genome," *Genetica*

On October 1, 1992, the day we first heard the words *fragile X syndrome* in the harshly lit office of Doctor #5, we were not the same family who had seen Doctors 1 through 4. The year and a half leading up to that day had been littered with a string of disasters among our families and friends. In March 1991, Harry's mother was diagnosed with terminal pancreatic cancer. An indomitable personality, Connie had only recently retired to live on a golf course in Florida, and she was not about to give up her life. She opted for an experimental chemotherapy treatment from Germany that took her hair but could not take her will. As she grew weaker and weaker, her dark Greek eyes shone out from her bald head with surprising beauty. She returned to St. Louis to die, and with the help of hospice care, morphine, and the frequent visits of Harry and his brother John, she was able to die at home, thirteen months after her diagnosis.

Cancer haunted this period in our lives. A month after Connie's diagnosis, in April 1991, my young cousin Steve lost his long fight with melanoma and died at age twenty-six. At the graveside, my uncle's grief was so raw that I could not bear to look at his face. A month before Connie's death, my father was operated on for colon cancer and began a year of chemotherapy. With characteristic stoicism, Dad attributed any queasiness he felt on the day of his weekly chemo to his pesky sinuses. My father had had cancer before (kidney cancer in 1978), but this second and unrelated cancer terrified me, maybe because I now knew how ruthless life could be. Around this same time, my best friend, only thirty-nine years old, had a routine mammogram and ended up with a mastectomy.

Harry and I were in our late thirties, but up to then we had not known life—or death—so intimately. Then, in late summer 1991, while his mother lay dying, Harry told me he wanted us to separate. To say that I was stunned is both true and untrue. At some level, though we had been together almost half my life, I knew we did not work well as a couple. We talked easily to each other, but only about the surfaces of our respective lives, not the secrets that fueled our dreams and desires. Still, my first reaction was to try to convince him that he was wrong, that we belonged together, that we just needed to reconnect. Though he seemed to have made up his mind already, I convinced him to try counseling with me. The doctor we saw together, a wise and seasoned psychiatrist, described me tactfully as "tenacious" in my grip on my marriage. I only gave in when Harry told me that he loved our son and would always love our son, but—and this he shouted, desperate to make me hear—he did not love me anymore. Like the last block in a child's tower, this piece of blunt truth collapsed my delusion that we would stay man and wife.

The story of our marriage has beginnings other than a rogue gene, not much clearer perhaps than the murky origin of my DNA, but it is a story line I will not try to follow here. When Harry's mother died the following April, it was only a few days before he moved out of our house, on the eve of his fortieth birthday. Now, five months later, we were sitting together in a doctor's office and facing a new, more serious diagnosis for J.P.'s problems. Doctor #5's "official" diagnosis for our seven-year-old son was PDD, pervasive developmental delay, and it was the most serious one J.P. had yet received. PDD is a behavioral disorder on the autism spectrum, affecting speech, communication, and social interaction and featuring repetitive, compulsive behavior. The three of us, still a tiny, provisional family, went out to lunch after the doctor's visit. Eating hamburgers and, as usual, trying to manage our son, Harry and I felt for the moment unusually close in our shared anguish. Having someone else recognize and name behaviors that had frustrated and at times overwhelmed us came as a relief, and yet this new diagnosis was deeply frightening. As J.P. grabbed at packets of sugar on the table and let out an occasional shriek, we saw and heard him as the doctor had that morning, as the others in the restaurant saw him now. We drew in closer to our son at the table and turned our backs on the room.

We didn't talk at all about the doctor's alternate diagnosis, this genetic disorder called fragile X syndrome. But something about the prospect that my genes and mine alone might be responsible for our son's problems resonated with my newly separated state. Sometime within the next two weeks I took a blood test, hoping to avoid a tussle between a phlebotomist and a writhing J.P. What I didn't know when I asked my internist to order the test was that a simple chromosomal test would only reveal whether I had full-blown fragile X, which I obviously did not. My doctor, like most medical professionals in 1992, was unaware of the recent advances in testing made possible by the discovery of the FMR1 gene. Carriers of the fragile X premutation could be identified only by more sophisticated DNA analysis.

In 1991, in those awful months while Harry and I and our loved ones had been living and dying, scientists had finally perfected the technology to test DNA for the unaffected carriers of fragile X. That discovery revolutionized detection of the disorder and allowed families to receive genetic counseling.

So it was that my chromosome study, begun October 15, came back eleven days later as a "normal female karyotype" with no evidence of fragile X syndrome. But a note reported in terse laboratory prose that I was "mosaic" for another chromosomal defect and should undergo a second round of tests. (Mosaicism occurs when two cell lines with different genetic makeups are present in a single organism.) I looked at a sheet on which were arrayed twenty-two pairs of bent little lines ranging from two inches to a quarter of an inch long; in the lower right corner was the sex chromosome, showing my X, an innocent inchworm no different to the eye than the others. This Xeroxed sheet, its cool duplication, felt like a violation of a sacred place; my chromosomes suddenly seemed as private as my uterus. I felt hot shame at the thought that my essence had been broken up into pieces and laid out on a slide. I was a "normal female," wasn't I?—but I was "mosaic for two cell lines." Mosaic. Cut into little pieces and set into mortar.

My doctor authorized the additional test, and on November 12 an amended report again ruled out fragile X but did find possible evidence of another, unnamed chromosomal abnormality. At the bottom, under "Recommendations," I read "Genetic counseling." I would later find out that the tiny percentage of mosaic cells reported in the test reflected either a technician's error or the fact that we all carry genetic anomalies of which we are ordinarily unaware because they have no impact on us. What strikes me today is that it was the recommendation to see a geneticist for an unrelated (and ultimately inconsequential) quirk in my genetic makeup that led to the discovery of the genetic bonds that forever link my son's identity to mine. I'm sure some doctor would eventually have tested J.P. for fragile X, but who knows how many more months, or years, we would have been in the dark?

In December, acting on the ambiguous results of my own blood test, I asked J.P.'s pediatrician to draw his blood. The holidays came and went and I put the whole matter out of my mind. Then, on January 21, 1993, as I worked in my study on a cold winter's day, the doctor called me at home. He gently told me that J.P.'s blood test was positive for fragile X syndrome. As I stared blindly at the icicles outside my window, I felt the blood rush to my ears. He explained that fragile X was a relatively common cause of developmental delay, accounting for 30 percent of X-linked mental retardation in males. No one had used these words before in connection with my son: mental retardation. He was retarded, a retard. My stomach lurched.

"How did this happen?" I asked. "My family is fine; there's no history of retardation." The pediatrician said that fragile X need not be inherited but could arise spontaneously. (At the moment this was a lifeline, but I would later find out that the odds of a fresh mutation were infinitesimal.) Clutching at straws, I asked, "Should Harry have a blood test too?" No, he had contributed only his Y chromosome to our son. In my attempt to share the blame for our son's condition, I had forgotten the most rudimentary high school biology.

When J.P.'s chromosome study arrived in the mail, I studied pictures of two slides of his blood. One looked a bit like mine, but the other was an array of stubby little blots; near the X chromosome a tiny arrow pointed to a puny tail on the blot, the fragile site. A third picture displayed a whirl of black rods, which to my untrained eyes looked random, ill-composed. It was another family picture—like my DNA study, like J.P.'s earlier CT scans—in a growing gallery of clinical abstract art.

A FEW DAYS LATER J.P.'s regular neurologist (Doctor #3) wrote me to recommend that I see a geneticist. He informed me, somewhat disingenuously, that my normal chromosome analysis did not rule out my being a carrier, a fact that I wish my internist and I had known earlier. The doctor went on to note that this diagnosis "does give us further information as regarding at least part of the origin of J.P.'s troubles, but doesn't change our approach to him from a medical standpoint." Of our seven-year-old son he wrote, "It obviously creates certain issues for him, ultimately, with respect to family planning. That is, however, years down the line."

There was no mention of family planning for his parents, who, though now separated, were still very much of childbearing age. In fact, not much more than a couple of years previously I had been convinced I was pregnant again and went so far as to write a whimsical Father's Day note to Harry from the child I was sure I carried. But that hope drained away in blood, unanalyzed, unread.

No mention, either, of my family of origin and the new families already created by my three younger sisters and my brother. Their situation would not be clear to me until March 22, 1993, when I met with a geneticist at Children's Hospital, on the same floor as the office of Doctor #3. He was another brainy, bow-tied, prematurely gray Harvard doc. I had a list of questions and he answered each one, meticulously and dispassionately.

But first he took a family history, probing for signs of intellectual deficiency in the previous generations. I could not help him there. My mother had had one cousin who was mentally retarded, but that had been due to oxygen deprivation during a difficult delivery of him and his twin. One of my sisters had a mild learning disability. One of my nieces was developing a bit slowly, but her problems were nothing so dramatic as J.P.'s. My sisters and I had graduated summa and magna cum laude from college. My brother, I boasted, had dropped out of college but had the highest IQ in the family. Defensive, rueful, anxious, argumentative, I defended my family's honor in the face of blood tests and statistics.

I learned some genetics. Each of us receives twenty-three chromosomes from each of our parents, the geneticist explained, on which all our hundred thousand genes are arranged like beads on a string (today we know it's more like thirty thousand). Fragile X syndrome is a single-gene disorder located on the X chromosome, the chromosome J.P. received from me when he was conceived. He was who he was before birth, the doctor assured me; his condition would not worsen, nor would it improve. Males with the condition are typically more severely affected than females, as they do not have the other, "good" X to supplement the "bad" X. The FMR1 gene (fragile mental retardation—that word again) makes a protein crucial for proper brain functioning, and in fragile X syndrome the gene suffers a mutation that shuts down the production of this vital protein.

The doctor said I was most likely what is called a carrier of the mutation. What is insidious about fragile X, and what had baffled the string of doctors we had consulted for our son, is that the abnormal comes from the apparently normal. Catastrophe is gradual: a stretch of DNA expands slightly in one generation, slightly more in the next, and finally reaches a breaking point in the third. The premutations are, for the most part, silent.

DNA is a sequence of four letters (C, G, A, T) standing for the nucleotides cytosine, guanine, adenine, and thymine. In a normal stretch of DNA on the gene called FMR1, the sequence CGG is repeated about thirty times, with a gray zone in the forty to fifty-five range: an unstable situation in which the carrier has no symptoms but there is a slight risk of expansion in later generations. An individual with a premutation, like me, would have fifty-five to two hundred repeats and a high likelihood that the mutation would expand in her children. Anyone with more than two hundred repeats is considered to have the full-blown mutation and would experience the effects of the syndrome, as J.P. does.

The doctor began to sketch a family tree, carefully drawing the males as squares and the females as circles. My son's square alone was blacked out. The tree extended only from the circle that was me; Harry's square sat unencumbered, irrelevant here because the only X chromosome J.P. had inherited came from me. Next to me my brother and three sisters were aligned, along with a square with a diagonal line sliced through it—my brother Gerard, born and died prematurely, the result of placenta previa— and a tiny black circle, the miscarriage my mother had not long after the premature baby.

On a faraway branch of the tree I saw my first cousins: one girl my age, one boy my brother's age, and their dead brother, a square dissected diagonally by a spot of melanoma. I thought of each of them, of the straight and oblique lines that held us all together. Tears rolled down my cheeks. The geneticist looked embarrassed. He pushed a box of Kleenex my way. "What's wrong?" he asked, somehow failing to see that his dispassionate lecture had turned my world upside down. I was just beginning to grasp the enormity of the diagnosis we had pursued for so long.

I had always been the one in my family to have an interest in genealogy. Five months later, almost to the day—in late August 1993—I found myself in the southwest of England, on a walking trip in Cornwall and Devon. I was trying to recover the person I had been before that time of devastating loss, setting off as a newly single woman to a country I had visited twice before, including summer study at the University of London. Always an Anglophile, preferring English to American literature during graduate school, I was also half English on each side of the family (the other half, just as beloved, was Irish). Strangely oblivious to the connections between genealogical research and my family's recent news, shortly before my departure I began to look up Dunsfords in the Boston-area phone books and through a couple of phone calls even tracked down Dunsfords in Prince Edward Island, Canada, where I thought my next trip might take me. My genealogical instincts were impulsive and scattered, but I was drawn by urges both new and ancient.

In the end I didn't really learn where our family had come from, but I was satisfied with making a special detour to the village of Dunsford while the rest of my tour group sampled the better known sights of Devon. I visited the fifteenth-century church and the graveyard, bought postcards of Dunsford at the post office, and had a Devon cream tea. What struck me most was that Dunsford consisted of just one main street, from which no side streets appeared to issue. The road stretched on and on, but as I stood there alone in the late summer sun, my eyes saw only a dead end.

# THREE

# Linkage

## *Family Ties*

The propensity of some characters (genes on a
chromosome) to remain associated instead of
assorting independently is called "linkage."

—Benjamin Lewin, *Genes VII*

I now knew how Pandora felt.

Designed by Zeus as punishment for the human race, Pandora was sent to earth, where she lifted the lid of a great pot and released all the ills in the world. Predestined for trouble—genetically engineered, you might say—she was an unwitting agent of disaster. Did her hand tremble as it lifted the lid?

Mine did as I lifted the phone to make the hardest phone call of my life. My parents and three of my four siblings lived in St. Louis. It was clear from my talk with the geneticist that I would have to explain to them the source of J.P.'s delays, that they were deeply implicated in this new diagnosis in a way that none of us could ever have imagined. The doctor had recommended that all of my siblings be tested to see if they were carriers of the fragile X premutation. A genetic mutation such as Down syndrome—typically a fluke of reproduction—descends on one child in a family, but an inherited genetic mutation like fragile X overspreads a family with grief, the effects expanding like a length of DNA stretched to the breaking point.

I am the oldest of five, four girls and a boy spread out over eleven years. As I contemplated giving my sisters and brother this news, I thought about its impact on each of their lives. One of my sisters already had two children who seemed to be normal, a girl of three and a boy of five. Another had a fifteen-month-old baby girl, whose development, unknown to me, was already a source of concern to her mother. A third sister was engaged to be married seven months from then. My brother and his wife were expecting a baby. Babies born, babies yet to be born, both the past and the future possibly blighted. . . .

My father and mother had both come to the phone at my request, perhaps thinking I had good news. I tried to picture them: Mom probably on the stool at the kitchen desk, Dad perhaps in his favorite wing chair in the living room. Slowly, haltingly, I explained J.P.'s diagnosis and what it meant for our family.

Dad broke into my explanation, his voice raw and quivering: "Damn it! They're not your 'siblings,' they're your brother and sisters!" I was used to Dad's temper, but this blast over the telephone receiver caught me by surprise. And yet, as I look back now, I can't blame him. I had been using the language of the geneticist, like a child unwittingly repeating the curse words of a nasty friend. My parents had agonized with me for seven years over J.P.'s failure to develop normally. Now they were being asked to consider that his problems were not unique, that my grief in Boston could be repeated four times over. It was too much.

As I explained what I knew of the genetics of fragile X, my father initially responded in the only way he could in the face of the unthinkable: with anger and disbelief. A law professor, he used the weapons of logic and skepticism to fight the diagnosis.

"How can you be sure this doctor is right? How reliable is this genetic blood test?"

Unable to answer that, I told him numbly, "He told me the odds of a carrier [*Yes, me, Dad, and maybe your other four children*] having a child with fragile X were fifty percent."

My father barked back, "Those are statistics! Anyone can manipulate statistics!" He slammed down the phone.

Stunned by this attack on the messenger, I spoke to my mother briefly and then hung up so they could digest the news. I sat shaking on my bed, trying to lose myself in the pink geometric pattern on the duvet cover. I had just broken my parents' hearts, but at that moment, sitting alone more than a thousand miles away, I collapsed into my own situation. I began to count my losses. Separated from my husband of fourteen years, I had now also lost my chance to have any normal children, even my chance for grandchildren. Who knew what losses lay in store for the sisters and brother I loved?

My father soon recovered his senses, and after his initial denial he consulted a geneticist—alone, by his own choice—to better understand the news I had given them. My parents were devastated, but we never spoke of our feelings as a family, not then and not now. My sisters and I speak one to one, but never when we are all together. My parents' support since that day has been largely silent: supporting their children through child care or money, contributing to the National Fragile X Foundation, witnessing our tears. In writing this book, I break that silence. I also hope to break the stranglehold of a linkage that grips our family like a clenched double helix.

MY SISTER ANN'S HUSBAND, James, was in medical school at University of Missouri in Columbia when we learned of fragile X, and he arranged for the family's DNA tests through a doctor he knew there. My siblings would be tested with the relatively new DNA test for the premutation, and their children would be tested for the full mutation. My blood had been drawn at my first meeting with the obtuse geneticist, and my DNA was now being analyzed at a laboratory in New York, though there was no longer any doubt that the test would show I was a carrier. I didn't know at the time what my family's expectations were, each one an actor in his or her own scenario, but soon after I had dropped the bombshell, my sisters Maggi and Cathy and my brother, Mark, drove the two hours from St. Louis to Columbia to have their blood drawn. Riding with them was Maggi's daughter, Meg, who at three must have seen this excursion simply as a family outing, a trip to her aunt Ann's house to visit her younger cousin Elizabeth.

This part of the story, like so many other parts, has always been a blank for me: what it was like for them to share the journey I had just traveled so utterly alone, separated from my husband; to offer blood together (the nervous laugh and averted head, the quick prick, the firmly placed Band-Aid); to break bread afterward, looking nervously at the familiar faces around the table (who would be chosen, who would be spared?). Did they remember me as they raised their glasses—me, the canary in the mine, whose passing from our old familiar life would either save them or doom them? Their oldest sister, the one with the hard-to-raise boy whose problems now had a name—would they end up like her?

My brother, Mark, has since written to me that, while he had assured his wife there was no danger for the baby she was carrying, inside his world was spinning. He wrote, "I desperately wanted to find out, one way or the other, what the truth was. One of the hardest things at the time was that Fragile X was an enormous dark evil cloud of undefined potential and painful reality.

"I remember joking with my sisters. And loving my sisters. What a strangely disparate crew of deeply beautiful women are my sisters. I remember thinking, 'Whatever this is, I love them and I see they love me.'"

Ann has told me that from the time she was a teenager, when she worked with children with cognitive and emotional problems at a summer camp, she had always had an intuition that she would give birth to a child with special needs. She went so far as to warn James when they were engaged that this was her future. So as Ann awaited the arrival of our siblings to her home in Columbia, she felt that the test they were going to take would simply confirm what she had always known. Along with her dread to meet her destiny was an odd feeling of excitement that Mark, Cathy, and Maggi were going to visit her apartment, which they had only visited once before, when Elizabeth was born. This blood-forged gathering was also a social occasion.

Mark described it this way: "There was a sense of all of us bonding, like performers in a play. A sense of 'us.' A sense of 'them.' Our wagons were circled." It must have been this fierce closeness that James later described to Ann, the sense he had of being an outsider when the group went out to a restaurant after the blood tests. The only non-Dunsford at the table, he marveled at the family sense of humor as my brother and sisters bantered over margaritas and appetizers.

"Well, this explains a lot," they joked, "about the Dunsford family!"

Ann felt it too, the bonding Mark described. However, back at her apartment, as the margaritas wore off, she told me, everyone was more somber, suddenly aware that if their feelings of closeness were sealed in the genes, there would be no turning back. Over the next couple of weeks my sisters and brother called each other, touching base as they awaited the results. I don't remember their calling me. Either Pandora had been exiled, or perhaps they thought my bad luck would be contagious. The first results would tell whether my siblings carried the premutation; the results of the children's test for the full mutation would take longer.

Ann was alone, the baby sleeping, when the doctor called on Holy Thursday of 1993. Her first words after the doctor told her she was a carrier of the fragile X premutation were "Does this mean I can't have more kids?"

The doctor paused. "Well, there are things you could do. We can look into them."

After they hung up, Ann walked into Elizabeth's room and stood over her crib. Ann had always dreamed of a large family, maybe six kids; now she looked down at this little blond girl and figured she would be her one and only. Elizabeth woke up then and, oblivious to Ann's tears, smiled to find her mother already at her side. Ann simply picked her up and held her tightly.

But more news was still to come, of course. This time when the phone rang, two weeks later, Ann took the call in the doorway of their little galley kitchen, as Elizabeth sat nearby in her high chair. "The test shows that Elizabeth does have fragile X," the doctor said quietly (the same doctor who had told Ann she was a carrier, so that Ann in her numbness apologized to her for having to give more terrible news, and on a Saturday no less). Through her tears she watched Elizabeth popping Cheerios into her mouth, looking calmly at her anguished mother as if the world had not turned upside down.

Fifteen minutes later the phone rang again. It was our sister Maggi, who simply said, "Do you want me to come down there?" Both of their little girls had tested positive for fragile X syndrome. Now the two of them, Maggi and Ann, cried on the phone together, with not a lot to say.

Later Ann called Cathy, who had also found out she was a carrier, but for whom the news did not have the same punch. Cathy was engaged to be married, but she had always felt that motherhood was not in her future. Her grief was more for the rest of us, though I have always wondered how she felt deep down about biology confirming her earlier instinct.

I wish I could remember how I found out that my sisters were also carriers. Was it a call from each of them? Did my mother tell me the news? Did I learn it piecemeal or in one crushing phone call? My mother also has a blank in her memory surrounding this period of revelations. She thinks each of her children told her their genetic status independently, but she isn't sure. While it has been more than a dozen years since this period of our lives, something else is at work in our family amnesia. Some things cut so deep that the pain obliterates consciousness—and strangles speech.

As if to underscore this mental whiteout, my journal never really records directly the blow of my family's diagnosis. What words I could manage trail off on the page, unbounded by end punctuation and followed by blankness: "Found out on Monday the implications of J.P.'s having Fragile X" . . . I would not write in the journal again for six weeks, and not about fragile X for three months.

Mark, the only noncarrier among us, felt he had lost a lottery of sorts, and in his relief over his unborn baby's future, he felt himself begin to join the group of "them," his sisters closing ranks in an "us" that no longer included him. He and I never spoke of these feelings until recently, when he admitted that it has hurt when, over the years, two of his four sisters have said, "You can never understand."

"Maybe I can't," he admits. "My heart tells me I can. But it's hard to show. I think the sharing of pain with nonrelatives is easier, perhaps." He hopes that as time goes on, more of the "us-ness" will return for him and his sisters. Our genes bind us and they tear us apart.

LIKE MANY LARGE FAMILIES, when we were kids we sorted ourselves into two groups according to physical traits or temperament, more like Mom or more like Dad. The brown-eyed group included those like Dad—Mark and I—and the blue-eyed group were those like Mom—Cathy and Maggi. When the fifth child, Ann, came along, rather than break the tie, she obligingly came with eyes a changeable hazel. Another sorting device was age and family order: my brother and I were the eldest, only eighteen months apart, but then my mother lost two babies in a row. When Cathy, Maggi, and Ann arrived, one every other year, they became "the Girls," a trio born after a gap of five years between my parents' first family and second. Gender put Mark in his own category, though in our family history and my own imagination, he was joined there by our lost infant brother, Gerard, who haunted my very notion of a brother. An interest in science and math put Maggi in her own category, along with her blond hair and freckles. The rest of us regularly teased her that she must have had a different father, for we all felt drawn to words, not numbers. So many varied ways to sort the data, and now this, this genetic sorting that we had not asked for: it seemed to cast sisters together and brother outside, based on an invisible number of repeats on a gene that threatened to sort the next generation too.

Six years after our family's diagnosis, Ann found herself pregnant again. From the moment she learned she was pregnant, she felt a deep tranquility, an overpowering sense of blessing. The baby might get the fragile X, but it could also get the good X; the odds were fifty-fifty. Somehow, though, Ann had faith that all would be well. The baby arrived without much warning, after a short and sweet labor, in the back of the family car, but Ann had chosen the name months earlier—Hope—for she believed that this baby was a gift.

Inevitably the doctor called again, several months later, with the news that Hope also had fragile X. Hope has proved to be only slightly affected, however, and like many girls with fragile X, could not be picked out in a kindergarten line as distinct from the girls next to her.

The next generation has been sorted in the genetic mainframe, and four out of six of our children carry the fragile X mutation. But they can be sorted in other ways, too. Two have dark hair, and four are blond. One has a talent for math, and the rest love poetry. Two are boys and four are girls. They are a "strangely disparate crew," like their parents.

FOR SEVERAL YEARS after Ann was born, when I was ten, I had a recurring dream in which I was saving her, the baby of our family. She was being chased by a bear, she was drowning, she was lost, and no one noticed but me. In the dreams I always rescued her. In the light of day, though, while I was the first to catch sight of the danger, I couldn't save either of us.

Did Pandora feel guilty when she saw what she had done? With the cagey ambiguity of myth, the story doesn't say. Me, I felt the burden of having lifted the lid on the troubles within, but I knew that eventually, under the sheer pressure of its contents, that pot would have exploded.

The story of Pandora has a happier, alternative version. When she replaces the lid, after all the troubles have escaped, something remains at the bottom of the pot—hope. It holds fast.

And, our family might add, it arrives in surprising ways.

# PART II

*Hotspots*

A hotspot is a site at which the frequency of mutation
(or recombination) is very much increased.

—Benjamin Lewin, *Genes VII*

It has been more than a dozen years since my family learned that
some of us carry a mutated gene on the X chromosome, and we
all began to rewrite history. My son was seven when I learned the
name for his developmental delay. J.P. is now twenty-one years
old, a boy ("Mom! Excu-u-use me! *Man!*") whose bright blond hair
has darkened to a sandy color, whose green eyes alter subtly with
the color of his clothes, a perfectly built five feet eight inches of
quirky humanity.

J.P.'s mother and father still love him with a fierce protective-
ness. He lives during the week with his mom, and on weekends
and some vacations goes to his father's house. His father still
takes him on road trips to the racetrack, listens to their favorite
country music together, and recently taught him to shave. J.P. has
a stepmother who helped him conquer his fear of dogs, and two
little half brothers and a half sister, as well as a golden retriever
named Wynonna, after his favorite singer. His mom is in love with
a man who laughs when J.P. tells the same knock-knock joke for
the sixth time and whose extended family love to have J.P. visit.

After being included in the regular elementary school with the help of a teacher's aide, J.P. attended a special-needs program in our town's middle school, mainstreaming in English and social studies. Today he attends a vocational program housed in a high school in a neighboring town. Recently he took an IQ test, which scored him in the mildly to moderately retarded range, but which did not do justice to a young man who correctly answered the question "Who wrote *Hamlet?*"

We have both been learning new things every day in the past dozen years or so, he and I—about each other, about the gene that helps to make him who he is becoming, about what is appropriate behavior ("Don't kiss and hug strangers"), about the depth of human kindness, about the way fear can paralyze, about how to tie a shoe, about the way grief ebbs and flows, about how to be proud of who we are. There are days we forget what we learned the day before, but we keep our brains on alert for what's important.

We're not alone in this brave new world. One in 3,600 boys has, like J.P., a full mutation of the gene that causes fragile X syndrome. One in 4,000 girls does, too. And one in 700 males and one in 259 females, like me, carry a premutation that can wreak havoc in the next generation.

Everything and nothing changed for me in 1993. My life fell into Before FX and After FX. I had to look back and see with different eyes my own past and my little boy's, and I had to re-imagine our future. Picture Victorian man compelled by Darwin's *The Origin of Species* to consider the idea that he was part of a world ruled by flux and mutation, bestowed with a kinship as brittle (and as fragile) as bones. Ideas take a while to sink in—the human ego has many defenses—but the force of an idea can upend a cosmos.

Yet even the seismic shifts caused by errant DNA cannot destroy some things. J.P. and I are more than just one gene. Even after fragile X, I still had these: an unquenchable belief that in and under life lay poetry; a constitutional hunger for order over chaos; a mother's blood-strong love for her child. X does not always herald the end of the alphabet. In the scrambled syntax of our new life, it is in some ways just the beginning.

# FOUR

# Replication Fork
## *Motherhood*

The replication fork is the region of DNA in which
there is a transition from the unwound parental duplex
to the newly replicated daughter duplexes.

—Benjamin Lewin, *Genes VII*

Him whom she loves, her idiot boy.

—William Wordsworth, "The Idiot Boy"

When I found out I was pregnant, in December of 1984, I immediately planned to keep a record. I had kept journals on and off
since I was nine, when I made cramped jottings in a locked five-
year diary about the weather and my latest adventure with my best
friend. Somehow, though, as if my new state didn't seem quite
real, I didn't begin my pregnancy journal until I was four and a
half months along. It wasn't until I first felt the baby move in my
belly that I began to write. It took the flesh to become word, you
might say.

"Quickening," I wrote, "what an expressive word for it—like a
pudding gelling, or milk turning to curds and whey, or the magical coming together of ideas in the writing process."

I was in the midst of a double gestation, for after years of ma-
lingering and months of false starts, I was in the home stretch of

my doctoral dissertation. As my belly got bigger, week after week, I pushed my chair a little farther back from my typewriter, but always pushed on, my due date a built-in incentive to finish up. "I feel so fruitful/fertile sometimes I could burst," I wrote in my journal. On its green leather cover were three stylized rosebushes, each of which bloomed out of a spiral shape that my eyes can't help but read today as a double helix.

Giddy in the creative process, I was grateful for the simple fact that where there had been a blank page, now there were words, not to mention that where there had been two people, now there were three. In fact, the former seemed more miraculous to one with writer's block than the latter. It is probably no coincidence that my dissertation studied a poet who was obsessed with the process of creation, a poet who suffered many dark nights in which he yearned for "the one rapture of an inspiration." Gerard Manley Hopkins, writing in Victorian England, lived in an age that throbbed with debates over when and how life began (as we do once more today). Clearly influenced by the debates over evolution, Hopkins imagined all change in the terms of his time: the catastrophic and the evolutionary, the abrupt and the gradual. A Jesuit priest, Hopkins preferred the lightning flash of creation by a divine hand to a slow emergence from anonymous slime.

In truth the moment of conception is less a moment than what is today regarded as an unfolding process. No one—no thing—really springs full-blown from its creator's head, an Athena from Zeus; there is always a story, a history, behind what's brought into being. J.P. was both engendered in a moment's union and looked for by eons of unfolding DNA. He came to being on August 8, 1985, and yet he came to being months and even years before, nascent in the wayward nucleotides that danced in my family's blood. ("Nine months she then, nay years, nine years she long / Within her wears, bears, cares and combs the same,"

Hopkins wrote of his mind, the fertilized "mother of immortal song.")

J.P. was coming to being in my head as well as in my womb during the nine months of his gestation. Somewhat self-consciously, I wrote in my journal at about four months along, "I've decided that the first three months of pregnancy are surprisingly (at least to me) physical, while the second trimester is more spiritual, a time of idealizing the baby. (My hunch is that the last two or three months return you heavily to the physical reality of it.)" I was always a bit of a Platonist, believing in ideal forms that never realized themselves on earth, though a part of me believed they would, like that Perfect Cottage on a Perfect Cove that I had seen in County Kerry in 1977. In the first weeks of knowing I was pregnant, my Platonic baby looked a lot like a little boy in a television commercial that played around that time; he was wide-eyed with a mop of brown curly hair like Harry's, and he wistfully lisped a song about wishing to be an Oscar Mayer wiener.

Later, as I felt the first random pulses of life in my belly, I tried to picture the fetus that was within: "When I picture the baby now," I wrote, "I picture it somersaulting in water, kind of goofy looking with a big head and closed eyes, endearingly clownish." This is a poignantly prescient description of the infant I was to have, in a way looking like all infants, but with the clichés intensified.

Later still, shortly before his birth, thanks to technology, I had a "real" picture of my baby, a black-and-white ultrasound rendering as unstable as an optical illusion.

"See his hand," Harry marveled.

"Oh, I thought that was his foot," I muttered. The first picture for the family collection was no less puzzling than the CT scan and chromosome studies to come, no more telling. In reproduction there is always the chance of error. A tiny smudge on the Xerox, a different angle on the paint stroke, a different intonation in tonight's performance—a mutation in a gene. Perhaps it's nature's way of ensuring uniqueness.

Writing this book, I asked J.P. one day if he knew what I was writing about. "*Moi,*" he answered with a glint of pride. It's all there: his surprising wit, a sense of style that defies IQ, but, most of all, the reminder that the J.P. I am writing about is a fictional subject, italicized as a foreign word. I can never reproduce the flesh-and-blood J.P. Though I once produced him, he was immediately lost to me, separated into the mystery of himself.

BY NOW EVERYONE KNOWS that DNA takes the shape of a double helix, two twisting strands of polynucleotides held together like a ladder by the bond formed between the bases. The two strands are mirror images of each other, pairs of complementary bases (C can only face G, and A only T), running in opposite directions. It's as tight and close-fisted a structure as you could imagine. Even when DNA replicates—and of course that is the way of life—it does so parsimoniously, cleaving itself into two strands but each instantly reforming into another duplex. Each daughter strand (for so they are called) holds on to one of the parental strands even as it forms a new strand in perfect apposition to its parent. Biologists call this semiconservative replication.

Part old, part new, wholly in sync with what has come before, the new double helix is like a model child, just who you expected, your mirror image. If DNA were a family, it would be more like the Brady Bunch than the Simpsons (at least when it doesn't mutate).

When J.P. slipped out of my body, I heard, "It's a boy!" It took a couple of minutes for this fact to take hold, for I had nourished a hardy belief that I would be the mother of a girl. I just didn't imagine myself in any other role, nor did those who knew me—

small-boned and traditionally feminine, preferring ballet to basketball, one of a family dominated by women. Of course, within weeks I could only fancy myself as the mother of a son. Looking into J.P.'s eyes, once he got used to keeping them open, I felt the bliss of completion. My mother said that she had never seen me so relaxed, so still, as when I fed J.P., our eyes locked.

Of course, my mother would know, wouldn't she? She knew me as a worrier, a perfectionist, an anxious little girl who tried to please adults. I was the type who got stomachaches on test day, the type who hyperventilated. In fact, the night before I gave birth, as I found myself unexpectedly hospitalized for the first time in my life while the doctors monitored my preeclampsia, I had a kind of panic attack. Harry had just left my room to go home, so I called my parents in St. Louis. I couldn't catch my breath, and, long-distance, with gentle reassurances, they literally got me breathing again.

But motherhood, I hoped, was going to calm me down, creating a new role for the neurotic perpetual student. Ph.D. in hand, I anticipated a couple of years of idyllic days with my baby, rocking him to sleep, crooning lullabies, later finger painting, building with Legos, exploring the zoo. But the serenity of feeding time was short-lived. Mostly J.P. cried a lot, and fretted, and tensed his body against mine as I held him. He always seemed on guard, a condition known as hypervigilance, which is one of the traits of fragile X syndrome, something I only learned much later. Loud noises, bright lights, crowded places—the stock-in-trade of contemporary life—overstimulated J.P. to the point of frenzy.

Like most of my generation, I had planned my pregnancy carefully and, once pregnant, treated my body as a precious vessel, avoiding caffeine, cigarettes, drugs, alcohol, even cat litter. So when we realized J.P. wasn't developing normally, my first thought was *What did I do?* Even a mother always blames the mother. I thought back to the night, before I knew that I was pregnant, when I had had cocktails and wine while out to dinner with friends. Then, at the end of the multicourse meal, a gourmand friend pressed me to order a snifter of very old, very expensive brandy. Now my baby was paying the price.

And then there was the old Victorian house Harry and I were renovating during my pregnancy. The sweet Hungarian man whose company we hired to paint the exterior took me aside. "Stay in the back of the house in the kitchen," he warned me. "That paint we're scraping has lead in it. It could hurt your baby." I did as he told me, but what if I had inhaled that poisonous paint and it had injured J.P.'s brain?

When I finally did learn that the source of J.P.'s problems was genetic, I was off the hook. Though in one sense I had caused them, in another sense I had done nothing wrong. I was not a bad mother, as I had feared. But what kind of mother was I?

CUT TO A DUCK POND in a leafy suburb, the pond adjoining a stately town hall. Dozens of mothers and their babies and children joyfully feed a flock of ducks and geese, pausing to sit on the park benches or picnic under the trees. One woman chases after a little boy about four years old; she can hardly keep up with him as he moves ceaselessly around the perimeter of the pond, stopping just for seconds to toss some bread on the ground inside the fence, on top of piles of other bread that will be left to rot by the overfed ducks. A large goose approaches the fence, almost as tall as the boy; it honks and jerks toward him as the boy shrieks and begins to cry. A fly buzzes by; the little boy shrieks louder, running away from his mother. He spots a flock of pigeons and darts into them, shouting incoherently. His mother talks continually, giving names to the things they see, the things the little boy is doing, but he doesn't talk back.

Around and around the pond they move, the mother talking, the boy shrieking, flinching at bugs and birds and geese, unable to stand for more than a second at the wire fence, fuzzy with caught feathers. He cannot pause to see the ducks nesting in the shallows, he cannot stay to see the crows stealing the bread, he barely looks as one duck skids over the surface of the pond in a comic landing; his eyes don't focus where his mother points. The mother looks at her watch, at the other mothers. It has only been fifteen minutes since they arrived. And now a dog bounds out of a car that has just pulled up. The little boy becomes hysterical and runs up the hillside. His mother follows, panting and defeated, wondering what to do to fill the next fifteen minutes.

WHEN J.P. HAD FINISHED the Early Intervention Program, Harry and I met with the preschool coordinator in our town and enrolled J.P. in his first Individual Education Plan: he would attend preschool in an early childhood multi-needs program. Not long after his third birthday, he traveled, a tiny figure in a yellow raincoat with a duck's bill on the hood, to a school twenty miles down the highway to get a battery of therapies and educational interventions to address his many delays. For the first few weeks, not yet trusting him to the school van, I drove J.P. to school myself, which also gave me the opportunity to observe his classroom. I still didn't know where my son fell on the spectrum of delays that demanded he be sent far from home to find others like himself.

The children in his class had fairly serious diagnoses: autism, cerebral palsy, pervasive developmental delay (PDD), mental retardation. One or two were in tiny wheelchairs, their limbs twisted or their faces askew. A couple of boys screeched instead of talking, as J.P. did. Most ran around in random patterns and moved with sudden jerks so that the classroom rocked and rolled like the deck of a ship on the ocean. J.P. was sometimes louder than the others, and he was even less able than his classmates to sit still for a game of duck, duck, goose. One minute I thought he should not be here (he looked so normal!), and the next minute I thought he was far behind his classmates in every way. (Why couldn't he stay in a line and follow the teacher?) A little piece of my heart broke off each time I visited his classroom, but in truth it was a place of love and ingenuity and patience, where J.P. got everything he needed.

I was now part of a "special" community too, whether I wanted to be or not, and this time I willingly participated in a weekly support group for mothers of kids who attended the CHARMSS Collaborative, a consortium of special-needs resources that served seven local school districts. Walking into these meetings was like walking into a steam room. Each woman was stripped bare; the air was thick with moisture, the voices disembodied. My mother has a theory that in the extremity of old age, we are just who we were in younger days, only more so. So I felt, as I looked around the circle at this motley assembly of mothers united only in bad luck, that I knew them as they were before the clouds of grief enwrapped them. Naked as they were now, I could still see them as they looked in street clothes, back when they blended in with the rest of the world.

One by one, we confided our stories. The mother of an autistic boy reported that her son had spat on her and struck her when she brought him to school that day, but her voice held no trace of anger; I recognized and loved her sweetness, and knew she was no different before this latest challenge. A woman told a tale of her child's birth, and of the moment she was told he had Down syndrome; I heard and almost saw her scream coloring the bleached hospital air and knew in my gut her hysteria. I knew she had always let her voice ring out. Another woman refused to curse the doctor who caused her son's cerebral palsy; she had accepted tragedy before. My own story, I was afraid, revealed me at my worst—impatient, perfectionist, unprepared by the smooth good luck of my past life to accept the adversity that had befallen me.

I seemed to choke up more than the others as I tried to put into words the ache of disappointment. And there was no name yet for my son's delayed development, so I could still deny that I belonged here with these women. They were strangers to me, and yet they were my sisters.

The idea that tragedy transforms and ennobles those it strikes persists on the strength of a half-truth. It always leaves its mark, but not always for the better. It is often said that God sends kids like these only to those who have what it takes to love them. Those of us who give birth to a child with special needs, that tired but useful euphemism, have the dubious distinction of being dubbed as special ourselves, by a kind of transitive property of divine selection. This takes on a sinister resonance when the child has a genetic condition and the mother is the carrier. How often have I wondered whether I was up to the task of being J.P.'s mother when I had some of the same traits that made his behavior so challenging?

When J.P. was about five, he and I flew back from St. Louis to Boston as we had so often during his short lifetime, after a visit with Harry's and my families. It was New Year's Eve, a day chosen for the chance that the plane would be less full and the flight more relaxed. Harry and I were having a dinner party, but since Harry had returned to his law practice in Boston days earlier, he was cooking for our guests, and all I had to do was arrive that afternoon and unpack. The flight ordinarily takes about two and a half hours west to east. That day snowy weather, air-traffic delays, and equipment problems conspired to trap us in the plane for seven hours, including a layover in Syracuse, where we were not allowed to leave the plane while it sat on the snowy tarmac. J.P. was at that time hyperactive, mostly nonverbal, and needed constant entertainment. I read him book after book, gave him snack after snack, and walked the aisle with him, trying all the while to pretend that the effort I was expending was not draining my every reserve of patience.

Eventually J.P. quite simply lost it—he screeched, he hit me, he smeared me with spit, he bit me—and I fended him off, all within inches of our seatmate, a man who was as desperately trying to ignore us as I was trying to be invisible. Finally, as we deplaned in Boston, released from our long ordeal, he turned to me and said, with awe, "I don't know how you do it." Of course, you do it because you have to do it. I walked off that plane wound so tightly that when I saw Harry, I said through clenched teeth, "Here, he's yours. I can't even be near him." We canceled our dinner party and I spent the last day of the year steeping in a hot bath, trying to reassemble the parts of myself that had been left on that plane.

At least flights with J.P., while necessary to visit our families, only happened two or three times a year. It was daily life that wore me down. Since J.P. got constant ear infections, we had to go to the pediatrician to have his ears checked and obtain antibiotics at least once a month. To allow the doctor to insert the scope in his ear, I had to hold J.P. on my lap and wrap my arms around him like a straitjacket, and that was only the beginning of my increasingly strenuous efforts to restrain J.P. for doctors' examinations. By the time he was in his late teens, when a female doctor tried to swab his throat for strep, he kicked me so hard that I staggered, and a male nurse was called in to help.

J.P. feared dentists even more than doctors. Because he couldn't tolerate my brushing his teeth or touching his mouth in any way, he was five before I mustered the courage to take him to a dentist. As I tried to coax him into the chair, J.P. flailed at me; moaning and babbling, he immediately attacked the dentist when he approached, kicking him and trying to bite him. The dentist, although he specialized in treating children, looked shocked and angry and sent us home without being able to catch so much as a glimpse of J.P.'s teeth. I didn't blame him for refusing to risk his fingers in my son's mouth; I hustled J.P. out through the waiting room, with its tiny chairs and primary colors, ashamed that my child and I didn't belong among the children cheerfully playing there. Another pediatric dentist wanted to restrain J.P. to work on him, but I refused to serve up my child like a trussed roast in the dentist's chair. J.P.'s teeth went uncleaned and unexamined for another five years, when we had him treated under general anesthesia in a hospital.

Because J.P. was unusually sensitive to touch—occupational therapists call it tactile defensiveness—even getting a haircut meant a nerve-racking session at a local children's hair salon. During these visits I stood by nervously as J.P. shifted continually in his chair, pulled off the apron, and tried to cover his head and ears, screaming and sometimes crying. Fortunately I found Karen, who, miraculously, never once drew blood as she wielded a scissors over the moving target of J.P.'s head.

Other aspects of J.P.'s sensory issues even affected our eating in restaurants. Until J.P. was about six he scooped up most food with his hands and smeared it on his face and the tray or table in front of him, the result of low muscle tone. Factor in his fidgeting and screeching before we had finished eating, and the stares from people at neighboring tables, and Harry and I eventually started leaving J.P. at home with a sitter when we went out. One by one, I crossed off the activities we could not do as a family.

I began doing all my errands—the cleaners, the grocery store, the drugstore—during the hours J.P. was in preschool, racing frantically home to meet his bus at 2:45, often pulling into the garage as the bus entered the driveway. I would anxiously help him down the steps of the van, gauging the rest of the afternoon by whether he was screaming or smiling and whether he stepped willingly into the house. Transitions of any kind were hard for him, even coming back home, where he wanted to be. I then became a prisoner in our house until the next morning unless I could hire a babysitter. I grew to dread holidays and teachers' training days, when students had the day off.

Shortly after my separation from Harry, in a quixotic attempt to share a normal childhood experience with my son, I bought tickets to the circus for one of those long weekends when we had nowhere to go. I must have been delusional. J.P. hated loud noises, as Harry and I had learned a couple of years earlier, when we were guests of friends at a country club in Florida on the Fourth of July; J.P. had screamed and covered his ears as the first explosions of fireworks burst in the sky. Despite all the evidence, I held on to my fantasies of what childhood was supposed to be: Platonic set pieces of picnics, pony rides, clowns. Ignoring what I also knew about my own weaknesses, I spent ninety dollars on tickets to the Barnum & Bailey circus at the Boston Garden, Boston's famous arena.

I normally avoided driving into downtown Boston because, having a terrible sense of direction, I tended to panic in the face of the winding and unmarked streets. The day of the circus, as nervous as if I were going to compete in a race, I picked up J.P. early from school to drive from our suburban town into Boston. Sure enough, I got confused as soon as I got off the turnpike and found myself snaking through unfamiliar streets, cars honking at me, my anxiety level soaring. In the back seat J.P. kept saying over and over, "I wanna go home." Sweating and cursing, I finally found my way to a multilevel parking garage, paid another twenty-five dollars for the privilege of parking there, and dragged him from the car.

Once in the Garden we pushed through the crowds, with J.P. occasionally swatting at people who bumped him. When we reached the section where our seats were located, my heart sank: they were up several rows, near the top of the stadium. J.P. hates heights and stairs of any kind, and even today he often ascends the stairs from our basement by bumping up backward on his bottom. These stairs were so steep that even I felt off balance. As we began to climb, he started screaming and shaking. I hissed at him to keep moving, desperate to reach those seats, but it was pointless. People were staring at us, and he simply planted his feet in the aisle. Defeated before the circus had even begun, I grabbed J.P.'s hand and headed back to the main concourse.

With tears stinging my eyes, I was just about to trudge back to the car when a kind security guard asked me what was wrong, and I blurted out my story. "Go to the business office on the first level," she said. "We reserve some seats for children with special needs." I told my story to the bemused person in that office ("No, he is not physically handicapped; he's just afraid of heights"), and he gave us seats right on the floor of the Garden.

I'd like to tell you that we settled in with cotton candy and J.P. was awestruck at the high-wire performers and tickled by the clowns, but that never happened. Being so close to the action totally unnerved him. The elephants' smell as they loped around the ring, nose to tail, repulsed him. The blare of the MC's barker voice and the screams of other children hurt his ears. We left within half an hour.

THE ROLE OF SUPERMOM, whether bestowed on me by friends or by strangers like my in-flight seatmate, lies heavy on my shoulders. A couple of years after the diagnosis, I spoofed it in a line of Mother's Day cards that I created for my own amusement with genetically challenged mothers in mind. One card shows a set of arms with bulging biceps: "On one of those days . . . ," it reads, next to a picture of human figures cowering under a monster, "just remember—you've got the X-tra strength it takes to be a mother." Another reads, above the picture of a spaceship, "X-traterrestrials recognize X-tra special mothers." I sent the cards to my sisters, but they weren't quite as amused as I was, and I never produced any more.

Two years after J.P.'s diagnosis, I attended a fund-raiser for fragile X research and met several other mothers of children with fragile X. Up until then, I hadn't met many women besides my sisters who shared in this unique motherhood. I was still deep in the weeds of adjustment, and my anger and bitterness at what had happened to my family dominated my better side.

As I stood near the bar, three of the women walked over to introduce themselves to me, a newcomer to these official events. Out of the blue, one of them smiled insanely and announced, "If this is the worst thing that ever happens in my life, I'll consider myself lucky." I whirled toward her. "This *is* the worst thing that has happened in my life," I said fiercely.

The truth is, my life had been pretty damn good before fragile X entered it: a protected, comfortable childhood, success in school, a large, happy family, the gifts of health and affluence. My life was pointed toward more of the same until I took the fork to motherhood. When I reproduced, I produced a cataclysm that swept over me and then my extended family.

"I love my son with all my heart," I protested angrily to these strangers, "but look at what all of this means—I'll never have more children, I'll never have grandchildren. How can you say this isn't the end of the world?"

"Well, I was depressed for about two years," the woman admitted, "especially when I accidentally got pregnant and had a second child with fragile X. But now the sun is shining again."

Feeling I'd wandered into a group of Stepford wives, I simply fell silent. Maybe it was my Catholic guilt, my sense that I should be an all-suffering mother, but I felt I was being tested by these women, interrogated about my own ability to accept what we shared, which was a natural disaster or a divine blessing, depending on our perspective at that moment in our lives. Of course, there were other aspects to all of our lives that played significantly into the way we experienced our child's genetic disorder: whether we had partners, whether we had other nonaffected children, whether our extended families also had children with fragile X, whether we had money or education—in short, many of the factors that can determine women's happiness all over the world.

At that moment, divorced only sixteen months, I felt keenly my single state; I felt as if I had a scarlet *D* on my chest. My divorce from Harry had been the other blow to my expectations of life, and, coming only shortly before I learned the source of J.P.'s delays, it had become intertwined irrationally with the idea of fragile X, one more in the cascade of terrible consequences that flowed from my reckless bite from the apple of knowledge. It was as if wife and mother had both been diagnosed, and I found myself banished from the world as I knew it. At the ticket table at the door at the fragile X event, I had been introduced to another parent, and besides relaying the all-important facts of my child's age and gender, I had blurted out that I was divorced. Without skipping a beat, the woman had asked, "Did the fragile X cause your divorce?"

"Of course not!" I had sputtered, outraged at the invasion of my privacy, protective of Harry, who remained (and remains) actively involved in J.P.'s life. But the question hung in the air. This woman would not be the last to ask it of me through the years. It would be silly to deny that a special child puts a special strain on a marriage, though it is difficult to come by statistics on divorce among people like Harry and me. Harry and I handled the frustration and disappointment of parenting a child who failed to meet our expectations in very different ways. I know it didn't bring us closer. But I honestly believe we were incompatible well before we had J.P. His problems made it more difficult to be partners but did not cause us to separate.

Standing alone at this fund-raiser, I envied the working partnerships of some of the couples at the party. One young couple had even switched places for a year, the husband taking a leave of absence from his teaching job and staying home with their very challenging son to give his wife a break from the stress of caring for him full-time. It was an arrangement unthinkable in my own traditional marriage, and yet they took it for granted. On the other hand, another woman there told me her husband worked twelve-hour days, leaving her as the sole caretaker of their two affected kids.

Another FX mom approached our group and, with mint-scented breath, shouted into my ear over the blare of the band, "Where does your son go to school?" If I were at a cocktail party in Wellesley, my hometown, this question would have very specific subtexts: Is he in an expensive prep school or in the public school? If he's of college age, is he applying to Harvard, Brown, or MIT, or to a state university? But my questioner that night was positioning us in a different hierarchy, no less important as we tried to fit ourselves into the world in which we had ended up. Her question really meant: Does your child attend school in a separate special-ed classroom or is he included in the mainstream? Does he have an aide or is he independent? *Is he more affected than my child?* is the whispered subtext, and I forgave her for asking. I wanted to know too.

As parents of children with a syndrome that causes mild learning disabilities all the way up to severe retardation, FX parents are simply trying to gauge our own child's place in the spectrum, not to mention the quality of our town's special services. The truth is that most males with fragile X are moderately mentally retarded, as my son is, and although assisted inclusion in the mainstream is the best setting for young boys with fragile X, they require more specialized and separate education as they mature.

And this is where motherhood spills over into the larger social space we inhabit. I couldn't raise my child alone. Every time we attend a team meeting for his Individual Education Plan, Harry and I are awestruck by how many people participate in the process of raising J.P. Speech therapist, occupational therapist, physical therapist, psychologist, teacher, teacher's aide, an occasional mainstream teacher: we are not alone in our love and care. It was J.P.'s gifted preschool teacher Pat who toilet-trained him. Did I feel displaced? Not for a moment. Even when Harry's new wife, Jaime, was the one who helped J.P. overcome his fear of dogs, I could feel only a deep gratitude. I haven't had the sense of "ownership" over J.P.'s development that the typical mother has in our culture, which uniquely exalts mothers without offering them a larger support system.

From the time J.P. was born, Harry and I employed sitters, first just for the ordinary Saturday night out but, later, when I went back to teaching part-time, for extended hours in the daytime. When Harry and I separated, I hired a live-in nanny for J.P., for the convenience and stability that situation could offer. Kathleen told me later that she knew the job was right when J.P., then age six but with the language of a two-year-old, ran down the hall to the room she was to occupy and placed his stuffed animals on her bed. Kathleen was a second mother to J.P. for nine years, seeing us (for surely I was her charge as well) through the difficult transition from family life to single motherhood.

The day Kathleen came to interview was one of the luckier days in my life. It can't have been much fun to live with J.P. and me in those first excruciating years after Harry left. I was in so much pain, eating little and sleeping poorly, and I wasn't used to living with someone who was not my husband, so I alternated between being standoffish and friendly with my new roommate. But

Kathleen was always cheerful and patient with both J.P. and me. She was a perfect alternative mother for my son: we were about the same age and each came from a large Irish Catholic family. She was articulate and vivacious and had lots of experience working with kids with special needs.

Sometimes I have felt through the years that because I had to depend on so many of these mother-substitutes, the Pats and the Kathleens, in order to raise my son, that I was a sort of mother manqué, the opposite of Supermom. Then, too, my experience of motherhood is so different from the typical mother's that when I used to listen to my friends talk about their children's normal activities and milestones, I would keep silent or mutter, "I don't know what that's like," disqualifying myself from the game. I was like a maiden aunt at a family reunion, unable to counter with family tales of my own. With time, I realized that my life as J.P.'s mother demanded to be told in the poetic, nonlinear style he favored himself.

I never imagined I would be the mother of an only child, but I effectively became barren on the day of J.P.'s diagnosis. I dared not reproduce again. All carriers of fragile X have a fifty-fifty chance of passing on the X with the premutation to a child, but since I am a carrier with a very high number of CGG repeats, there is an almost 100 percent chance that if a child receives my fragile X, it will expand to a full mutation. Though the diagnosis came just as I was separating from Harry, I had not ruled out a new life and more children, and that dream died in an instant. The irony is that J.P. is able to bear normal children. A male with fragile X syndrome passes on his Y chromosome, which is totally normal, to his sons. Interestingly, his sperm cells have only the premutation, so his daughters are only carriers, women like my sisters and me.

But the odds are that J.P. won't reproduce. Though fragile X syndrome does not affect his fertility, his social and cognitive deficits and the way his nervous system becomes overwhelmed will likely deter him from consummating his sexual feelings. In one way, this is a relief to me, as clearly J.P. is not capable of caring for a child. On the other hand, it fills me with grief to think that he will never know the intense pleasure of sexual intimacy or the gift of his own child. Now that he is a young man, J.P.'s hormones are definitely in overdrive. He speaks of girlfriends, and sometimes talks of marrying one day. The extent to which J.P.'s romantic notions will become reality I just don't know. I hate being the guardian of his sexuality and can't escape the irony that this is just what I struggled against in my own parents. I don't have the luxury of allowing my son to express his sexuality in the way I wanted to at his age, not for the religious reasons my parents invoked, but for the blunt fact that J.P.'s brain is not as developed as his penis, and never will be.

The FMR1 protein seems to regulate hormones, and its absence in those with fragile X syndrome results in oddities of their reproductive systems. Most males with FX have enlarged testicles, especially once they have passed puberty, a condition called macroorchidism. (Seeing one of my sisters change her infant son's diaper, I thought, *Well, he sure doesn't have my son's equipment!* I had no idea at the time that her son was built normally and mine was not.) Some females with the full mutation have enlarged ovaries or enter puberty early. And some women with the premutation experience premature menopause—POF, a medical acronym for premature ovarian failure. The fragile X phenotype is an odd mix of hypersexuality and sexual deficit, the organs larger than normal but the chance to reproduce diminished—nature's cruel joke.

X IS A CHIASMUS, a place of crossing where two things meet. I am constantly confronted with the complex ways in which J.P. and I mirror each other in our own necessary and close-held bond.

More than once, when I drove J.P. to his elementary school, I watched as he stood stock-still on the top of the hill leading down to the playground, which swarmed with a hundred little boys and girls weaving in and out of playground equipment, four-square courts, hopscotch grids—the intricate geography of childhood. J.P. would pace right and left, trying to find an entry point, trying to catch the rhythm of the dance. He would step forward and immediately step back. In kids with fragile X this is more than social shyness; it is the experience of being overwhelmed by the sensations that a chaotic scene induces. This would go on for four or five minutes. It was as excruciating to watch as it must have been to live in his body: shut out, aching to be let in, your nervous system tripping you up so that your feet couldn't go where your brain directed them, where your heart was flying. As J.P. hovered on the edge of his schoolmates' turf, I sat in my car, nervous and self-conscious, watching the other mothers chat outside the school, making playdates and comparing teachers. His isolation was mine, too.

Like J.P., I have trouble with transitions. My family didn't foster fresh starts or new horizons. For better or worse, we do not like change. This is not a matter of genes but is more like a fossil of family patterns that have their bedrock in Irish patriarchy and English insularity. My maternal great-grandfather, known as "Papa" to all in the Meehan family, refused to come out of the house to say good-bye the day his youngest daughter, my great-aunt Catherine, moved from his house with her new husband. He could not accept that his daughter wanted to leave his home. My paternal great-grandfather, known as "Father" even three generations down the line, lived in the last years of his life with my grandmother Bumbie and the wonderful man she had married when my grandfather died, and I had the sense as a little girl that when push came to shove in my grandmother's affections, Father would come before her husband, Bert.

My own parents lived within walking distance of their parents, and my siblings live within five miles of my parents today. My leaving St. Louis for graduate school in Boston and then settling down with Harry here has put me outside the borders of the Dunsfords' closely drawn map. Sometimes I can't believe I did it, unwound the coils of the blood bond and spiraled off a thousand miles away.

Yet I have re-created a familiar configuration, the parent and child who cannot cut the cord. Would it have been different if J.P. were a typical child? So much has conspired to draw us together, perhaps a bit too tightly. Since Harry and I separated when J.P. was six, the two of us, mother and son, have been an unholy dyad, embedded in our home without family nearby or the friends that a typical child would have to draw him away from his family. J.P. has social instincts but does not have the social skills necessary to maintain friendships. I myself am extroverted but also a loner in many ways, often preferring solitude to company. As J.P. matured, he romanticized me; I became his love object, an extravagantly praised creature who is mother, wife, all women in one. Though I now am in a serious romantic relationship, J.P. is slow to distinguish the love of a mother for a child from a woman's love for a man.

"Who's cuter, him or me?" he asks.

I answer, "You're the cutest son in the world, and Stephen is the cutest boyfriend in the world." He likes this answer, but still, a day later, the question comes again. The usual jealousy of a son of a divorced mother is amplified and distorted when your mother is the center of your universe well past the time when school, sports, and friends should be.

The crux of our exaggerated closeness though is the cursed fact that J.P. is deeply dependent on me. A man of twenty-one, he still has difficulty in buttoning his pants and starting a zipper. I still cut his toenails and clean his ears. I so often have to manage his behavior rather than gently guide it. I tell him when to brush his teeth and remind him to use toothpaste, tell him to wipe his bottom, tell him which side is the front of his shirt. They call it personal management in his special-needs classes, but it is supposed to be his task, not mine. I hate who I am in these moments when I try to control him. I am the subject to his object, when I want him to be his own subject. I hate the distance between us that comes from the lack of distance between us.

It is not just physical intimacy that accounts for our bond, though. J.P. has always had a kind of radar about my moods, picking up my anxieties and joys with the intensity of one whose nervous system twangs with each breeze of emotion. Even when he was five years old, if I cried, he would run to get me a tissue.

I remember a day when J.P. was four and we were visiting Grandma Connie in Florida. We had gone to the beach and J.P. had played in the surf, buffeted by waves in the hot sun. As he and I sat in the backseat on the way home, he leaned against me, letting all his weight go into my side. I suddenly realized I had never felt him relax like this before; his muscles were usually tense, and his body in motion. As I sat there in that hot car, my son's body melted into mine, I felt a sharp sense of what we had missed, the natural everyday feeling of being at home in the world and with each other.

The first summer that J.P. went to overnight camp, a place for special-needs kids in another state, two hours away by car, I relived the visceral agony of every childhood separation I had ever felt. Though he was almost seventeen, I could not imagine his living with strangers, far from my control. Who then would make sure he was clean, his clothes right side out? Harry valiantly agreed to drive him to camp and I would pick him up two weeks later, for we both knew I simply could not handle leaving him there. On the way back from Connecticut, Harry called me, shaken, from his car. He had left J.P. sobbing in the dingy cabin; he was equipped with a phone card though he didn't actually know how to use a phone. The next day I answered the phone and, after a young counselor explained that J.P. wanted to talk to me, heard my son's desperate, quavering voice: "Mo-o-om? Come get me! Ple-e-ease, ple-e-ease!" I have never felt so desolate, my chest tight with panic. I tried to calm him, to calm myself, and eventually he hung up.

"What do you think? Should we go get him?" Harry asked me when I reported the call. Everything in me wanted to rush to his side and gather him up, but I knew we had to give him the chance to do what he needed to do—to be in the world without us.

"No, let's give him more time to adjust. The camp director said I could call as much as I wanted to find out how he was." I did call, twice a day, over the next couple of days, and finally I was told that he was no longer crying but proudly keeping the cabin schedule on its clipboard. On the third day J.P. was crowned Camper of the Day. It took me another three days to unclench my stomach, to begin to savor the simple pleasure of being alone.

Biologists call the ability of DNA strands to unwind from the double helix denaturation or melting, oddly gentle terms for the instant when the base pairs are disrupted momentarily, wrenched apart from their primitive bond. When the two complementary strands reform into a double helix, it is called renaturation. Harsh and necessary as an infant's first breath, the ebb and flow of DNA creates the rhythm of life.

ONE OF THE ODDEST POEMS ever written is William Wordsworth's "The Idiot Boy," a long ballad composed extempore by the poet "in the groves of Alfoxden" in 1798. Critical reaction was mostly negative, at least in part because of the subject of the poem; idiocy violated poetic decorum in every respect. "Many feelings which are undoubtedly natural . . . are improper subjects for poetry," harrumphed a critic at the time. It is hard to describe "The Idiot Boy," as its narrative continually slides under a stream of nonsensical language: questions, repetitions, alliterations, colloquialisms, contradictions. With a "hurly-burly" and "a long halloo," the ballad gallops along gaily, ignoring conventional expectations of pace, direction, and sense—much like the idiot boy. Indeed, the idiot boy *is* the poem. Perhaps that is why, again and again, the narrator cannot find the words he needs to tell his story, for, in the end, it is not his.

> *I to the muses have been bound,*
> *These fourteen years, by strong indentures;*
> *Oh gentle muses! let me tell*
> *But half of what to him befel,*
> *For sure he met with strange adventures.*
>
> *Oh gentle muses! is this kind?*
> *Why will ye thus my suit repel?*
> *Why of your further aid bereave me?*
> *And can ye thus unfriended leave me?*
> *Ye muses! whom I love so well.*

With annoying repetitions and contradictory assertions that always threaten to overthrow sense, the narrator manages to stutter out the story of Betty Foy, whose "very idle" decision to send an "idiot boy" on a nighttime ride to fetch a doctor to save the life of her ailing friend Susan Gale begs the question, you might say, of who is the idiot. The narrator comments critically, "There's not a mother, no not one, / But when she hears what you have done, / Oh! Betty she'll be in a fright." Betty decides to lay a staggering burden of trust on the boy "who is her best delight" because she has no one else to turn to; her husband is off at work, a "woodman in a distant vale," a familiar story for many mothers.

At various points, Johnny is mute or he speaks in riddles or he "burrs," but, as a speech pathologist would say, he apparently has receptive language, for when his mother sends him off, she assumes his understanding as she rattles off a lot of advice. Her bossiness is understandable, at least to me:

> *And Betty o'er and o'er has told*
> *The boy who is her best delight,*
> *Both what to follow, what to shun,*
> *What do, and what to leave undone,*
> *How turn to left, and how to right.*

Betty lets him go, her idiot boy, against all common sense, and he returns her confidence not by doing what she sent him out to do—for he falls off the map of everyone's cognition, leaving a hole in the story, as no one (including the poet) can imagine where he might be all night long—but by being himself, by following his own course and still accomplishing the purpose of the mission, which was to restore Susan's health. For in her concern for the missing boy, Susan rises from her bed and "As if by magic [is] cured."

The moral of the story? Trust a mother's intuition? Fools are truly wise? Love cures all? All of the above? One lesson is that Johnny is who Johnny is. "You've done your best, and that is all," Betty says when she finally finds him. He has the shimmer of the ineffable about him, our silent Johnny, and the glamour of a romantic hero. He doesn't need to act to be effective; after all, a poem does not mean, but be.

> *Who's yon, that, near the waterfall,*
> *Which thunders down with headlong force,*
> *Beneath the moon, yet shining fair,*
> *As careless as if nothing were,*
> *Sits upright on a feeding horse?*

*Unto his horse, that's feeding free,*
*He seems, I think, the rein to give;*
*Of moon or stars he takes no heed;*
*Of such we in romances read,*
*—'Tis Johnny! Johnny! as I live.*

It is Johnny's story that rules the day. Johnny's unique perception of the world transforms a ride in the moonlight and the hooting of owls to its mirror image, but his version stands as the definitive one, trumping the narrator/poet's and, for that matter, the reader's. The poem ends as Betty asks for an accounting from her son: "'Tell us, Johnny, do, / 'Where all this long night you have been, / 'What you have heard, what you have seen, / 'And Johnny, mind you tell us true.'"

*And thus to Betty's question, he*
*Made answer, like a traveler bold,*
*(His very words I give to you,)*
*'The cocks did crow to-whoo, to-whoo,*
*'And the sun did shine so cold.'*
*—Thus answered Johnny in his glory,*
*And that was all his travel's story.*

It is not the exquisite triumph of night over day, the idiot over the poet, being over meaning, that moves me most sharply in this poem. It is the drama of separation and reunion, the mother taking the risk of letting go her boy, and the miracle of his return. Indeed, three quarters of the poem is devoted to Betty's complicated relation to her son, her love and pride growing to distress and even suicidal anguish as she fears Johnny has come to harm. Nothing would have been accomplished had Betty Foy not let her son go from her on his quixotic quest, his midnight ride as brave as his emergence from her womb. Life happens when the unitary bliss of one cleaves into two. It is the only way.

AS HIS LANGUAGE DEVELOPED, J.P. himself was able to express the desperate binary of our bond. Once, after I had yelled at him, age fourteen, for writing on his bedroom wall, he scribbled a note to me and slipped it under my study door. I called him in and, holding up his gibberish, asked sternly, "What does this say?"

Instantly, he replied, "Dear Mommy, You are a stinking jerk. Love, J.P."

Sometimes J.P. will come up the stairs from the basement in the home the two of us share, and I tease him by asking, "Who's that?" as if I were expecting someone else. He says indignantly and with inexplicable earnestness, "Mom, Mom! It's me, your daughter!" I have not yet figured out why he says this. There is much I haven't figured out about my son. He surprises me again and again, with who he is and who he is not. Like me and not like me, he is everything I could not imagine and so much more.

# FIVE

# Base Pairs

## *Like Mother, Like Son*

The genetic information in all living things is stored in DNA, which is present in chromosomes. Adenine, thymine, guanine, and cytosine (A, T, G, and C) molecules make up the DNA. They contain coded information that is required to construct a living organism and to direct the way it functions. The sequences of these four bases, A, T, G, and C, determine how you differ from other individuals and from other living things. The bases are paired, A with T, and G with C. We often use the term "base pairs," since the presence of the base A presupposes the presence of a T on the other side of the DNA molecule.

—www.fragilex.org

—Where art thou gone my own dear child?
What wicked looks are those I see?
Alas! alas! that look so wild,
It never, never came from me:
If thou art mad, my pretty lad,
Then I must be for ever sad.

—William Wordsworth, "The Mad Mother"

I've set up my laptop in my town library today. The sun is stream-ing through the windows and reflecting off the computer screen so that I can't make out a word. It doesn't matter, though, because there is nothing written there. I've been sitting here for an hour, paralyzed by the weight of my memories, my brain scattered with the dense acronyms that litter my life: DNA, RNA, FMRP, FX. Anyone else would simply call it writer's block.

But I am haunted by something that other writers don't carry: a mutation that has been numbered, pictured, and stored in my medical file. I carry 110 repeats of a sequence of bases spelled CGG on a gene on my X chromosome in a spot where the average person carries about thirty. Another ninety of these uninspired little phrases and I wouldn't be able to write these words, or, for that matter, to read them. I would suffer all the maladies J.P. suffers.

At noon I give up the struggle with my keyboard and go downstairs to sit on a bench in the library's lobby and eat my sandwich. Suddenly a gangly young man exits from the door to my left with two feather dusters in his hand. He gazes intently out the front door of the library, but turns left and disappears from view, only to emerge again empty-handed and go back into the library. It is my eighteen-year-old son.

J.P. goes to a special program housed in a high school in a neighboring town. The TEC Learning and Vocational Center places its students in volunteer jobs in various settings, with an eye toward discovering their future vocational placement. This year, his senior year in high school, J.P. works twice a week for two hours in the children's section of this library. I knew he was here today, but seeing him out in the world, unaware of my gaze, I have a startling sense of the future. After lunch, I peek around the corner where he had gone before. The door says CUSTODIAL CLOSET. I walk back upstairs to resume my writing. Somewhere on the floor below me, my son is dusting the books.

WHEN J.P. WAS FIRST DIAGNOSED with fragile X syndrome, and I realized that it came from me, not his father, I tried to summon up guilt, but found myself verbalizing something that frankly I didn't feel. I know a lot of fragile X mothers feel guilty for having passed on this gene to their kids—I've read heart-wrenching admissions of this on the Fragile X Listserv—but I've never let myself take on that burden. I feel I'm a victim of this as much as J.P. It's not like I snorted cocaine while I was pregnant, or knowingly worked at a hazardous job. All I did was conceive him, and that was enough to set into motion the tumbling unfolding of DNA that did us both in.

Seven months after the diagnosis, I wrote my father a letter trying to articulate how I felt about the notion of guilt. My parents did not get tested at that time, as our family history didn't seem to require that we discover the source of the mutant gene. My mother is an only child; my father has but one sister, and her children—my cousins—and their children seemed perfectly normal. However, all signs pointed to my father as the source of the mutation. That is because my brother, Mark, who had received a Y chromosome from my father, was the only one of the five of us spared the premutation. My three sisters and I, who received an X from each parent, were all carriers. I worried that my father felt a burden that he should not have to bear in addition to a grandfather's natural grief at his grandchildren's fate.

In the letter I assured him that blame was the last thing on any of our minds, my sisters and I. "The glory and the harshness of genetics is that there is no picking and choosing," I wrote to my law-professor father, my intellectual role model. "We are a composite, with all that means for success and failure, health and illness, strength and weakness, joy and pain. I look at J.P. and yes, I see his disabilities, but I also see talent, charm and character that also came in that genetic package. I look at myself, and, while I grieve over my reproductive damage, I am much more than a potential mother. Some of the things I like best about myself, that

I take the most pride in, come from *you,* Dad, your genetic contribution to my identity."

But what I didn't count on as I wrote this letter in October 1993 was that, with J.P.'s diagnosis, I would be tarred with the same brush. No sooner was the DNA test for fragile X carriers discovered in 1991 than scientists were off and running to investigate whether these carriers showed differences from their normal peers, whether they were "affected," a word I can never look at in the same way again after our diagnosis. And it was *our* diagnosis, not just J.P.'s but his three cousins' and, yes, mine and my three sisters' and one of our parents'. That's the peculiar heartbreak of the fragile X diagnosis; it is not unique to the proband, as they call the first person to be investigated in the genetic study of a family. It's contagious.

Eighteen months after fragile X entered my family's vocabulary, when J.P. was almost nine, two of my sisters and I attended a conference of the National Fragile X Foundation, a biennial event that draws researchers, medical personnel, and parents from the United States and many other countries. We were determined to learn all we could to understand this complex and devastating condition that had ravaged our family. In June 1994 the conference was held in Albuquerque, New Mexico, where Maggi, Ann, and Ann's husband, James, flew from St. Louis and I flew from Boston. At that time Ann's daughter Elizabeth was two years old and Maggi had two children, a six-year-old boy with no mutation and a four-year-old girl with the full mutation. Maggi and I shared a hotel room, so I spent most of my time at the conference with her.

Maggi was starting medical school in the fall, so she was particularly eager to attend the sessions geared toward scientists and doctors. I was interested in these too, though I had never taken any science in college except "biology for poets." At a lunch break on our first day at the conference, we strolled through a large meeting room hung with posters. One of the posters announced a study of carrier females.

"That's us," I exclaimed with surprise. The researchers had set out to investigate whether females with the premutation suffered a higher rate of depression than their typical and non-FX peers. And guess what? They did.

"Duh," Maggi and I said to each other. Raising a child with fragile X made you depressed. Gee, that was a no-brainer. We walked on.

BUT TO TELL THE TRUTH, that poster hit a nerve. I had received the news that J.P. had fragile X syndrome just eight months after Harry and I had separated. Since that time, and even as I dutifully took notes at this conference, I had been gradually unraveling.

I come from a Catholic family in which divorce is almost as serious a sin as murder. My parents had supported me unquestioningly in my pain over Harry's decision to end our marriage, but I felt as if my life would never recover from the shame of losing my husband and disrupting our child's life. Although in the eighteen years that I had spent with Harry, as girlfriend and wife, I wasn't happy in some basic way, I didn't have the insight or will to change my life. I had numbed myself to earlier dreams—of writing, for instance—even though Harry had never discouraged me from pursuing them. I do not blame my husband; I blame myself entirely. I was hiding out from life, afraid to try my hand at success. Shortly after Harry's leaving, I began to see a therapist to push my way through the tangle of feelings that overwhelmed me. Talking about the sudden changes in my life was clarifying and liberating, but if my mind was enlightened, my body didn't get the message; it betrayed its allegiance to other codes.

I wasn't sleeping well. J.P. went to bed at seven thirty on weeknights, and on the weekends he went to Harry's. I was alone night after night in our huge house on a cul-de-sac. The summer of the fragile X conference I found myself staring out the window of my upstairs hall one hot night. In the dead suburban silence a bird called out—a species I couldn't identify—and his mate, for surely it was his mate, called back. It went on for minutes, this eerie and beautiful call and response. I knew that no one would answer my call on the dark, deserted street. My family lived in St. Louis and I had few friends nearby, and almost none who were single, as I now inadvertently found myself. I ate little, and with a logic as inexorable as the genetic verdict I had received, the pounds dropped off me till my bones showed.

If the separation from Harry broke my heart, combined with the string of deaths and illness that had plagued our families around the same time, the visit to the geneticist the following March set the pieces in stone. That day I lost all hope of future children and grandchildren. On December 8, 1993, when Harry and I went to court to finalize the divorce, I didn't see how things could get much worse.

You could say I got my depression the old-fashioned way: I earned it. I didn't inherit it, or at least that's what I thought.

When I read that poster on depression in fragile X carriers, in a hotel in Albuquerque, I was, to all eyes, a vivacious, plucky single mom, educated, in control of her life. My writing students at Boston College the following fall surely thought so; their course evaluations touted my enthusiasm and upbeat personality. Yet behind this persona, in the still center point of my contracting world, a woman wept. At home, away from the university, from friends and acquaintances, I would collapse at the end of the day, tired of smiling and talking. I would put my child to bed, fix a Manhattan, and when the phone rang, I would sit in the dark, unable to pick up the receiver. I was crying many times a day, I was extremely irritable with J.P., and I felt hopeless. My therapist was attempting to convince me that I would benefit from antidepressants, but I resisted, stubbornly believing I could do this alone.

Heading for the big four-oh on my birthday that September, I racked up one more of the Top Ten Major Life Stressors I had seen listed in women's magazines when I moved, on Labor Day weekend, from the house Harry and I had shared into a new, smaller house. Before the move I sold all the baby furniture I had hoarded in the attic over our garage, a virtual storeroom of yuppie consumption: the crib, the swing, the changing table, the playpen, the walker, the high chair, the car seat, the rocking infant seat. I would not be needing any of these again.

It all came to a head in the hardware store. Scrambling to set up a house for J.P. and me and our two cats, overseeing painting and repairs, I went one day to buy new shades for J.P.'s bedroom. I asked a tall, ruddy, white-haired salesman if he could cut me a shade the same size as the one I held in my hand. "Not today," he said mildly. "The machine is down." With that, I began to cry. As the tears ran down my cheeks, he looked panicked, bewildered. I turned and ran out of the store.

That night I looked at myself in the mirror, and my eyes were flat and dead. My spark was out. I made the appointment, and on September 19, 1994, I saw a psychiatrist to get a prescription for antidepressants. I was depressed, and I was a fragile X carrier. But was I a depressed fragile X carrier?

WILLIAM WORDSWORTH, the great poetic investigator of feeling, wrote his *Lyrical Ballads* in 1798 to "follow the fluxes and refluxes of the mind when agitated by the real and simple affections of our nature." In "The Mad Mother" and "The Idiot Boy," two of his deceptively simple ballads, he set out to trace "the maternal passion through many of its more subtle windings." The mad mother is a homeless woman whose husband has deserted her and their baby. Her grief has driven her mad, but her passionate love for her baby saves her from throwing herself over the cliffs into the sea. Mother and child are a symbiotic pair:

> *The babe I carry on my arm,*
> *He saves for me my precious soul;*
> *Then happy lie, for blest am I;*
> *Without me my sweet babe would die.*

Her greatest fear is that she has passed down her madness to her son, and she strenuously denies her part in his "wildness": "It never, never came from me."

Where does the mad mother end and the idiot boy begin? This question, it turns out, intrigues many of those men and women who research fragile X syndrome. In any genetic diagnosis, it is natural to turn to the oak after you've examined the acorn. But that tree is not just a maker of acorns. It is shade and rustle and the silhouette of limbs against a winter sky. The oak may be oblivious to the human eyes that define it (the botanist's or the artist's), but a woman feels those eyes on her face. She either blushes or she raises her head in defiance and walks on.

AS THE CONFERENCE CONTINUED, Maggi and I began to get hints that we who went to the conference as mothers were seen by those who researched fragile X as carriers, and some of them suspected we were not immune from the effects of the premutation. Maggi and I often split up and went to different sessions— she to Molecular-Clinical Correlations and I to Why Does My Child Do the Things He Does and How Can I Help Him?—but at some point we were sitting in the same session when a group of women in the back of the room began to joke about what they saw as their carrier traits, such as a short attention span and not being good with numbers. This was the first we had heard of these cognitive manifestations of our new identity, and we were aghast. Focused on how to help our children, we were not prepared to see ourselves as impaired.

That night back in our room Maggi turned to me. "This explains it!" she squealed. "I have ADD! I can't keep my mind on what I'm studying!" I was appalled, but also a little amused.

"Don't even go there," I said with emphasis. "For heaven's sake, you graduated with honors from college; you're starting medical school. You manage a household and two children. You couldn't have ADD. We are okay! There is nothing wrong with us."

In fact, in 2003, researchers in the Netherlands concluded that a subgroup of female premutation carriers does perform poorly on several selective attention tasks, but they note that research on whether or not the FX premutation is associated with a particular neurocognitive phenotype has been "equivocal." That word sums up the ambiguity of my sisters' and my situation. Looking for signs of difference in people like us, members of the FX research community have conducted dozens of studies on carriers, both female and male, but have come to differing conclusions. While there is growing evidence that a small minority of carriers suffer some learning differences and subtle emotional problems, the samples studied are often small and the data contradictory. Words like *anecdotally* and *persistent reports* crop up in the scientific literature, betraying the elusive nature of the facts in this area.

A case in point: one in five women will suffer depression at some point in her lifetime, according to the National Mental Health Association. That is why it is important to be leery of statistics gleaned from studies in which a few dozen carrier women are examined for their incidence of depression. One study, in 1994, looked at four groups of women: two control groups without fragile X, one of which grew up in an FX family and one which did not, and two DNA-positive groups, one with a premutation and one with the full mutation. There was no difference among the groups in terms of lifetime incidence of depressive and anxiety disorders. On the other hand, a study published in 1996 examined thirty-five mothers of children with FX (twenty-nine of whom were premutation carriers) in comparison to two control groups: thirty mothers of children in the general population and seventeen mothers of autistic children without FX. They found that premutation carriers had a higher frequency of affective disorders than mothers from the general population, and—cognizant of Maggi's and my observation that raising a kid with FX could indeed make you depressed—the researchers note that the age of onset of psychiatric morbidity was much earlier than the age when the mothers discovered their child's special needs, so the burden of raising such a child could not account for the threefold higher frequency of affective disorders that they found in carriers.

I was unexpectedly introduced to another of the affective disorders under scrutiny in carriers when, in May 1995, Harry and I flew with J.P. to Colorado, to the fragile X clinic at Denver Children's Hospital. Apart from the fact that Harry flew the three of us in first class, it was a painful trip in every way. The larger seats and the extra service couldn't make up for the fact that when we got to the hotel, we checked into two rooms, J.P. and I in one and Harry in the other, the connecting door between them the only marker that we had once been a family. The awkwardness and careful politeness that now marked our relationship was the price of what Harry and I knew was a lifetime of necessary cooperation when it came to J.P. Fortunately, our love for our son has cemented a relationship grounded in years of shared history.

We made this long, expensive trip because we wanted our son to be seen by Dr. Randi Hagerman. In Albuquerque the year before, I had met Dr. Hagerman and many of the team of professionals she had gathered around her at the clinic in Denver: genetics counselors, occupational and speech therapists, educators, psychologists, all working in the field of fragile X, expertise we simply hadn't found in Boston. Denver was the mecca for fragile X families at that time, and Randi, as all the FX families called her, was its goddess. (Indeed, at a fragile X conference years later, Maggi and I saw her get in an elevator surrounded by her handsome husband, Paul Hagerman, a molecular biologist who also studies FX, her two children, and her elderly parents. Maggi turned to me and chuckled, "This is too much! She's not only brilliant and beautiful, but she's good to her parents, too!")

Dr. Hagerman is a developmental and behavioral pediatrician, a skilled clinician who radiates affection for those individuals with fragile X. Harry and I watched with delight as she examined our son, who was running away from her, refusing to look at her, flapping his hands and barely intelligible. She clearly got J.P.'s sense of humor, and she took in stride all the behaviors that had flummoxed other doctors because she had seen hundreds of other boys just like him. It was a relief to be, finally, in a place where we could get answers about a condition that usually was met with "Fragile *what?*"

Randi charmed me, too, that day with her observation that many of the carrier mothers she had met she had found to be unusually articulate and verbal. But she also mentioned a study that had found an increased level of worrying in carriers. I resonated with this particular trait, remembering how, even as a child, my mind worked on overdrive when I was faced with a new situation.

After we left Randi, Harry and I sat down with Louise Staley-Gane, a genetics counselor in the clinic. For the second time in my life I saw my family laid out on a genetic chart. This time Harry's family was also surveyed—father, mother, brother, each with any particular diseases they had suffered: cancer, psoriasis—but with my family the notations seemed to target psychological foibles. Though my father had had cancer (twice, at that point), the only notations next to his name besides his occupation, law professor and labor arbitrator, concerned his tendency to worry and his quick temper. My sisters and I also were labeled according to whether we tended to worry. Besides being a worrier, I confessed to mood swings and recent depression. Harry's notations said simply "lawyer" and "high blood pressure." Wasn't I a college lecturer with a Ph.D.? But maybe that wasn't relevant here.

Suddenly Louise asked me, "Can you leave the dishes in the sink after dinner, or do you feel like you have to jump up and wash them?"

Startled, I thought about it briefly, and admitted, "Well, I'm no great housekeeper, but I guess I do feel compelled to do the dishes right after dinner." I sat there uneasily, all too aware that my former husband was sitting beside me. Suddenly the diagnostic gaze was on me, not on our son. Louise was only doing her job, but the questions made me self-conscious. How about my fingers, she asked. Was I double-jointed? Sheepishly, I pulled back each thumb in turn; they popped out at a right angle to my hand. Feeling mildly freakish, I wondered, not for the first time, how I had ended up in this place—literally and figuratively.

Having hyperextensible joints is not exactly the end of the world. They come in handy for yoga, for instance. But another physical feature of some 16 to 25 percent of carriers is premature ovarian failure, or POF—in laywoman's terms, early menopause. My first thought when I heard of it at the Albuquerque conference was that this sounded like a good thing, although, a dozen years later, as I pass through that stage myself, I realize the havoc menopause can wreak on your body.

As coincidence would have it, one of the women who cared for J.P. after school a couple of years ago is a fragile X carrier and has a nephew with fragile X. One day I came home from work in a particularly foul mood and said casually, "Boy, do I have PMS!"

77

Maria didn't answer, so I went on, "How about you? Do you ever have days when you feel like you want to murder someone?" She paused.

"No," she said quietly, "I don't get PMS. I went through menopause at twenty-two." At that startlingly young age, she had had to take hormone replacement therapy and suffer the gamut of what menopause can do. She was devastated too, because it meant she could never have a child.

Besides premature menopause, the premutation is alleged to do other things to the carrier body, occasionally blossoming in long faces or prominent ears, traits that individuals with the full mutation sometimes have. Maggi and I once took our kids, not long after our FX diagnosis, to see a re-release of Disney's original movie *Snow White and the Seven Dwarfs*. Looking at Dopey, his tremendous ears flapping, Maggi turned to me and snickered, "Looks like a missed diagnosis." We had imagined that we were Snow White. Were we now bidden to check under our hair for Dopey's ears? (And why look that far? In 2003 a study was published that analyzed the hair roots of carriers as predictors of cognitive functioning.) This is not to make light either of the pathos of our children's impairments nor the exquisite investigations of dedicated scientists. It is—with the black humor that sustains my sisters and me—to speak for the amoeba under the microscope. Call it an unexpected blurt of sentience from the presumably inert.

In his junior year in high school J.P. mainstreamed in an honors English class, with the help of an aide and an extraordinary teacher. When the class studied Shakespeare's *Othello,* they put on a skit and gave J.P. the nonspeaking part of the dead Desdemona. He lay sprawled dramatically on the floor, but when the boy playing Othello forgot his lines, my son sprang up, the corpse come to life, and shouted the words that his honors classmate could not remember.

Do you know what it feels like to go through your life seeing yourself as a top student, the life of the party, the subject who views the world on the terms she sets, only to wake up one day to find yourself the object of a scientific gaze? This is not the same as being a patient, examined physically for an emergent medical problem. It is to find your past rewritten and a shadow cast over your present—to have your every behavior, your every mental process, scrutinized for pathology.

When I first heard these suggestions about carriers, I was only a year and a half from J.P.'s diagnosis and newly divorced after spending half my life with one man. I was not prepared for any more assaults on my identity. Clare Dunsford had become Clare Manion had become Clare Dunsford again. Suddenly I was asking who really was Clare Dunsford at thirty-nine, and for that matter, who had she been at nineteen, or nine? Was it possible that I had some incipient version of the syndrome my son had?

In the terms of the evolutionary debate that fascinated Gerard Manley Hopkins, my dissertation subject, had the catastrophe in my family really been sudden, or had it been gradual, sneaking up on the new generation in the unmarked moments of the old? Memories flood in, cast in a different light: the little girl who made herself sick with worry over gym class in grammar school, the teenager whose moods swung up and down so much that her journals seem to have been written by Ms. Jekyll and Ms. Hyde, the young woman who struggled both to start and to complete that doctoral dissertation.

Hopkins was drawn to brood long and hard over his own identity. As a child he asked, "What must it be to be someone else?" It is the ultimate mystery, this question of what sets me apart from everyone else. Where are the boundaries that make me perhaps neurotic but not insane, not a genius but not mentally retarded? Are they found in a set of numbers counting a stretch of base pairs? Is there a threshold of abrupt change at two hundred repeats, or as the chain gets longer does it drag, ever so gradually, on a person's brain?

The questions I ask are only possible in the wake of Darwin, who claimed the living world for the principle of gradual change. DNA is the fuel that drives that change, its mutations the pathway to variations in species. Genes are digital, not analog, agents, discrete nubbins of information, each with its own idiosyncratic power. However, the effect of genetic knowledge has been to elide originality and individuality in favor of a tendency to find identity in those who have come before you. It is the threat that Darwin posed that made Hopkins so concerned with settling the problem of identity once and for all in favor of originality. As a young woman, I had been led to study the influence of evolutionary concepts on Hopkins by an affinity deeper than I knew: a romantic predilection for uniqueness and a religious belief in miracle. Now, in my own crisis of identity, I resisted a theory of myself as one in a line gradually devolving toward extinction.

The most recent research on fragile X carriers operates on the assumption of a genetic continuity that results in a spectrum of involvement, with the full debilitating symptoms arising in the full mutation but some hints of them found in some of those with the premutation. The hypothesis is that the amount of FMRP—fragile X mental retardation protein—produced by those with a higher number of repeats is diminished, creating some of the impairments of those with the full mutation, who produce no FMRP at all. Interestingly, current research on autism, a disorder related to fragile X in some of its symptoms, is also focusing on its presentation along a spectrum of severity, with parents of autistic children showing some subtle autistic-like traits, presumably caused by shared genes. Autism is now thought to be caused by a complex interaction of several genes, possibly in combination with environmental factors. My child did not appear out of nowhere but was looked for in the genes that I passed on. While the number of wholly genetic syndromes is so far relatively small, in the brave new world of genetics, we will increasingly be forced to ask whether a diagnosis applies to us as well as our children. The truth is, I can't figure out if my mind roams around more than yours, or if my writer's block is some sort of deficit in executive function caused by my DNA. I have no point of reference. Like Hopkins, "I taste *self* but at one tankard, that of my own being." I do not know what you feel like when you write or worry or feel anger. I can only know our effects in the world, you and I: the books we write, the words we say, the feelings we elicit in those around us. The effort it takes to achieve those effects is usually invisible to the observer. It's fair to say that life is challenging for both you and me, but probably in differing and highly personal ways.

What I do know is that we are more than our DNA, more than what we "carried" into the world. We establish our identities in concert with others at the level of the family, the school, the city, the nation, the world. Nurture presides over us along with nature, and seasons the self that we taste in ways we could not have imagined at birth. I am made of my mother and my father, and my grandmothers Nanny and Bumbie, but I am also the creation of my childhood best friend, Mary Ann, and Sister Mary Stephen, the first-grade teacher who taught me to read, of the St. Louis humidity and the study tour of Europe I took in high school, of the moon landing and President Kennedy being shot, of the men I've loved and the poems I've studied, of yesterday's quarrel and today's embrace.

My sister Ann, after the diagnosis of her older daughter, worked for a time in the Frank Porter Graham Child Development Center in North Carolina, one of the leading centers in the United States for research on fragile X. Ann, like Maggi, graduated from college with honors, and has a master's degree in school and child psychology. Besides being highly intelligent, she is vivacious, beautiful, and has a steady, strong temperament. You'd trust her with your life. She told me that she was once at a meeting with the staff of the clinic when they began to talk of carriers' characteristics in clinical terms. My sister suddenly felt self-conscious, as if her competence were being questioned. Of course they weren't talking about her specifically—when she left the job to spend more time with her daughter, the clinic begged her to stay—but she felt the sharply uncomfortable feeling of being categorized. And for what? For a gene on her X chromosome that if she had not had children would never have come to light.

Is it hubris to resist being labeled? If it is, I plead guilty. Not every carrier resists the label. Some welcome the sense that their idiosyncrasies, their particular learning styles, have an explanation. Some can erase a kind of survivor's guilt that plagues them for having passed this gene to their children by seeing themselves, too, as somehow impaired. All of us who are FX carriers have to navigate this passage in our own way, and support each other in the effort. As the years have passed and I've made some peace with fragile X, I have become more ambivalent about its influence on who I am. While I resist it as a defining label, at times I take pleasure in the ways in which this fact about my genetic heritage seems to excuse some of what I'd like to disown: relentless worrying, a volatile temper, a vulnerability to sadness.

In the end we who carry the carrier label can gain compassion for what our kids must feel when they're objectified as "fraggles," not to mention acquiring a hard-won humility in recognizing that we all—you as well as me—"carry" a ragtag bag of characteristics that mark us as human. Some of our baggage carries identification tags, and some of it does not. As Louise Staley-Gane told me that day in Denver, everyone has six to eight genes that are potentially problematic. I just happen to know the name of one of mine. Maybe one day you'll have a name for yours.

FOR A FEW YEARS I thought that, like the "Mad Mother," I would be "for ever sad." The weight of what I carried pulled me down, "the heartless simplicity of the CGG repeats" (as Matt Ridley puts it in his dazzling book *Genome: The Autobiography of a Species in 23 Chapters*) carved in the stone of my heart. I could not deny my son's "wildness" came from me, that without C there could be no G, but I could chafe against the tightness of the bond. I began to push back, and in my resistance I began to find myself again.

While we were in Albuquerque, Maggi and I took a side trip to Santa Fe, a welcome respite from clinical descriptions of our children and ourselves. The clear yellow light and the glittering blue sky left us pleasingly disoriented as we wandered through a Native American outdoor market. Eventually we went into a building, climbing the stairs to a second-floor arcade, surprised to find ourselves slightly breathless in the unfamiliar altitude. In a gift shop there, I was attracted to a note card with a picture of a weeping woman: "La Llorona," it said on the back, "a Hispanic legend." I bought the card, and when I returned to Boston I sent it to Maggi with a note telling her how glad I was that we'd had the opportunity to share the conference together. I ended by saying, "Of this card—the Weeping Woman—I just want to say that I hope that we can give over our tears to the life-giving project of raising our children, not drowning them, with all the love and strength we can muster in the years ahead."

La Llorona's identity is a contested one, though I did not know it at the time. She is the heroine of a southwestern folktale, probably originating in Spain, who appears in many guises. In most versions of the tale, La Llorona is a beautiful young girl who is betrayed by a man and drowns their children in revenge or in frustration—the Mad Mother, if you will. In various accounts she appears as either murderer or victim, witch or innocent young girl, harlot or virgin. What endures in every telling of the tale is this: La Llorona mourns the loss of her children. Her apparition, with its keening cry, haunts the banks of the river.

One thing I must have sensed: she is my sister. And, yes, she is I.

# SIX

# Transcription
# and Translation

## Speaking of Love

A two-step process decodes the genes in DNA into
proteins, according to the **central dogma**. First, DNA
is copied into RNA (**transcription**). Second, the RNA
message is converted into protein (**translation**).

 —Sandra Pennington, *Introduction to Genetics*

The motive for metaphor, shrinking from
The weight of primary noon,
The A B C of being,

The ruddy temper, the hammer
Of red and blue, the hard sound—
Steel against intimation—the sharp flash,
The vital, arrogant, fatal, dominant X.

 —Wallace Stevens, "The Motive for Metaphor"

The reading has already started in the mahogany-paneled library
of this house on my university's campus, so I slip in quietly
and perch on the ledge of the built-in bookcases. I assume my
professional listening face—eyes trained on a distant spot, lips
pursed, eyebrows slightly lowered, hand to chin. The author, a

plump young woman, is reading a short story in a minimalist style, cute and glittering and laconic. This style has the same effect on me as *i*'s dotted with circles or hearts. Shifting on the hard wooden ledge, I can't seem to lose myself in the story.

I'm in a cranky mood. About an hour before, Kathleen, who has now been caring for J.P. for three years, has called my office.

"I thought you should know," she begins. "J.P. says his mouth hurts."

"Why? What's the matter?" I say, somewhat impatiently, as I am in the middle of a conference with a writing student. "Did he say how he hurt it?"

"Well, no." She hesitates. "I've asked him why and he can't really say. He even got some ice out of the freezer to soothe it, but I can't see any sore or blood in his mouth."

I begin to offer possible scenarios: Could he have bitten his tongue while eating his after-school snack? Might he have fallen down and bitten his cheek? Could he have a fever blister? Not that she knows of. He seems to be eating, and, aside from being a bit droopy, he is otherwise okay. Feeling nonplussed, I hang up the phone.

The writer is still reading her story at the podium. Her clear, plummy voice carefully enunciates the short, simple sentences sans transitions that are apparently a hallmark of her style. Wanting to give her the benefit of the doubt, but irritated by what seems a gratuitous obscurity, I find my mind wandering again to J.P.'s enigmatic pronouncement: "My mouth hurts."

ONCE AGAIN I am reading my son. All parents must occasionally read between the lines when their children speak, but my reading skills are more challenged than the average parent's. For me the space between the lines is the difference between, say, a single-spaced manuscript and a triple-spaced one. Even as the many doctors we consulted over seven years attempted to diagnose J.P.'s developmental delay, the primary symptom noted in their reports was always the delay in his speech. Or maybe that was just the symptom I first complained of when they asked why we had come to them. It was the silence that was killing me.

A passionate talker from an early age myself, I laved my first-born with words as I changed him and bathed him, as I fed him and held him, as I kept intimate company with him on those endless, lonely days of early motherhood. But the kinds of communication promised in the baby books never arrived. J.P. never babbled; he simply cried. He cried a lot. During the first two months he cried in pain from colic, and after that he cried at the pain that light, air, noise, and movement could cause his preternaturally alert senses.

And when he cried, I held him and rocked him. Our Victorian house had a curved oak staircase to the second floor that was punctuated by a broad landing, a space so generous that Harry and I once had a string quartet play there for a party. But on a daily basis the staircase landing housed our stereo and speakers, and it was here that I set up the rocking chair, backlit by the window, and looking out over the downstairs front hall as from a stage. Harry had an old album of Johnny Mathis songs that I had discovered soothed J.P.'s nerves, and so I sat in the rocking chair, playing Johnny at full volume, crooning over my little boy as he sucked furiously on a pacifier and gazed at me with the blind trust that I could ease his pain. A nimbus of golden oaken light surrounded us, mother and child, as the melodramatic vowels of "Wonderful! Wonderful!" rolled from top to bottom of the house. I have never felt so close to anyone, and I have never felt so all alone.

The months passed, and though his nervous system settled down a bit, J.P. neither babbled nor spoke. For that matter, he had just begun to crawl at almost twelve months, the age most babies begin to walk, when Harry and I rented a house on Cape Cod for the month of August 1986. One of the earliest home videos shot with the camera we so eagerly bought when J.P. was born records our son's first birthday party, held in the kitchen of the house we rented in Falmouth, Massachusetts. In the video, my sister Ann, who had come to visit from St. Louis, sits near J.P.'s high chair, talking to him, while visiting friends and their three children mill about; but all I can hear when I play this tape is the shrill voice of a mother who knows something is wrong. It makes me long for the silent home movies of my own childhood. Then no one would be able to hear my nonstop commentary as I speak for my son, the first of many times (as indeed I do here).

A home movie from my own childhood features me at about age five, chattering away happily in a strawberry-print bathing suit with a ruffled skirt, standing next to a plastic swimming pool while my younger brother, Mark, standing inside the little pool, silently fills it with a hose. In the unintentionally comic way of silent film, I prattle on for many minutes, hands gesturing and face moving expressively, my monologue as steady as the hose, the words now as lost as water down a drain. All the while Mark is dreamily filling the pool, oblivious to his big sister's chatter, unable to get a word in even if he wanted to. I like to think that the little girl who speaks with such animation is unaware that that there is an audience beyond the moment, happy just to entertain her father as he holds the heavy fifties movie camera and records this everyday moment of family life.

But in 1986, a new mother, I am all too conscious that Harry and J.P. and I are setting down a piece of family history in this video: I am filling the air with words not for the joy of it, but because my little boy cannot. I am desperately trying to concoct a scenario fit for a photo album—label it "Baby's First Birthday Party"—but the starring actor is not ready for his role. While the average one-year-old usually speaks three or four words and can jabber pretty good imitations of sentences, my one-year-old is seen in the video sucking silently on his pacifier or regularly letting out piercing shrieks. As the camera pans over the party, J.P. does not know how to play with the toys I unwrap for him and lay on his high-chair tray. I hit the keys of a tiny piano, and he cannot imitate me. Although he chortles and smiles in obvious delight, his body is utterly rigid, legs straight out and kicking, arms fluttering constantly, eyes blinking. On the floor toddles the one-year-old son of our friends; calm and centered, he looks the camera in the eye, plays the little piano, and says, "Look a' me."

On his second Christmas, when J.P. was sixteen and a half months old, he finally gave me the gift I had been waiting for. On a visit to his grandparents in St. Louis, as we sat around the tree opening presents, he called me "Mama." At least I think he did; it was close enough that we all agreed to call it that, the love-struck parents and grandparents who heard it—close enough to fill my eyes with tears. Up until then J.P. had had what pediatricians call "nonspecific sounds," including "dada," but no real words. Of course, he didn't say "Mama" again in any meaningful way for the next few months. J.P.'s baby book records that he said his first real word on April 8, 1987: *cookie*. He was twenty months old.

A few months later, in the fall of that year, I was reading a section of the *Boston Globe* quaintly called Confidential Chat, in which anonymous writers, mostly women, asked for advice and traded recipes. I saw a letter from a mother asking whether she should be worried about her two-year-old daughter who wasn't speaking yet but loved books and letters and seemed bright. This child sounded a lot like J.P. Hoping to share my fears, I immediately wrote to the woman, signing my letter with the pen name "Chatterbox." In reply, she generously mailed me copies of letters she had received from other mothers, all of them promising that things would turn out all right. Apparently their silent babies had all grown into healthy normal children who never shut up. These other mothers had been where I was, and had come out on the other side. For the moment, I decided I was one of them.

But as time went on, I grew to hate those developmental milestones in the child-raising books. Somewhere between fifteen months ("baby says a two-word sentence") and twenty-four months ("baby says a three-word sentence"), the reassurances of family, friends, and strangers began to stick in my throat, and I made the first appointment with a pediatric neurologist. It would ultimately take four neurologists to change the diagnosis in the chart from the plain and simple description "language delay and attention deficit" to the esoteric designation "fragile X syndrome."

WRITING ABOUT J.P.—I am quick to admit it—is easier than raising him. In the first two and a half years of his life I did not work outside our home, but eventually I missed teaching and adult companionship, and I took a job as a part-time adjunct lecturer at Harvard, teaching sophomore English majors. As I backed my Honda out of the driveway on the first day of school, I felt only one emotion: giddy relief. Maybe my mother was right: being a mother and running a house is far more difficult than studying Keats, at least when you feel you do the latter a lot better than you do the former. I was heading as fast as I could back to the life I knew and loved: reading and interpreting literature, and sharing that knowledge with college students. Karen, the Wellesley College student who cared for J.P., tried to make him wave from the kitchen window, but as I looked up, he was screaming and flapping his hands in a way that said not "bye-bye" but "fragile X," though at that point we did not have this phrase in our vocabulary.

Today as I search for the words to articulate my experience as a mother, to describe the essence of my son, it seems natural to turn to poetry. The climactic closing lines of Wallace Stevens's poem "The Motive for Metaphor" reverberate with a new meaning since J.P.'s diagnosis. "Desiring the exhilarations of changes," Stevens generates a dizzying list of metaphors that reminds me that the mutable and the mutant are linguistic cousins. In my attempts to make meaning out of the mixed-up alphabet that spells my life as J.P.'s mother, am I "shrinking from / The weight of . . . the A B C of being"? But if metaphor is my defense against brute reality, it is also utterly necessary. In the end, the only way to speak of some things—the sublime things like love, or joy, or sorrow—is in metaphor: "The vital, arrogant, fatal, dominant X."

"Fragile X" is a double metaphor, its name suggesting a weakness on a chromosome, identified by a letter that is, among other things, a potent metaphor for the unknown. It is a perfect metaphor for the breaking point of a life, and yet also for a crossroads at which to imagine a whole new direction.

Genetics itself is deeply saturated with metaphor. DNA has been imagined as a language for as long as the bases—the four chemicals that pair up to form the twisted ladder of the double helix—have been assigned letters, a deeply unexamined discourse that has led to the exalted evocation of the human genome as the Book of Life. In this light, you might say that any genetic disorder is a kind of linguistic problem. My son then becomes a kind of poorly written text, the extra CGG repeats clogging the sentence on the FMR1 gene a piece of verbosity that any good editor would excise. But the mutation alters the meaning of this text in a more basic way: beyond mere verbosity, it produces nonsense. The protein that the gene should make goes missing, and with it, the meaning of it all.

Like his hard-won diagnosis, with its oddly metaphorical name, J.P.'s utterances are often elusive and riddling. Some might call them incoherent, but I delight in their Dadaist ingenuity. One night after dinner, when he is fourteen, J.P. is scribbling at the kitchen table. He does not look up, but he knows I'm there. "She always gets my drift of negative boldness," he says, astonishingly.

I wait, holding my breath, to see what he'll say next. Still without looking at me, he dashes off another line, announcing with a bouncy lilt, "She had me as a baby. She always gives me lunch of salad and Doritos." A budding Beat poet is writing a tribute to Mom, right here in my own kitchen.

The very fact that J.P. speaks at all is a miracle to me. Around the same time that I went back to teaching, he began to attend the Early Intervention Program that I had at first denied he needed. He was assigned a speech therapist whom Harry and I began to call Eeyore, after Winnie the Pooh's donkey friend, for her lugubrious ways and pessimistic comments. Utterly lost in this new world of disability, one day I asked Eeyore the kind of direct question that you later learn not to ask: "Will he *ever* talk?"

Without a moment of hesitation, she said bluntly, "We just don't know."

I could hardly believe he would not, for J.P.'s favorite toys from infancy were books; I read to him constantly, and the books he liked I read over and over, like Sandra Boynton's *Moo, Baa, La La La!*

"A cow says, 'Moo,' a sheep says, 'Baa,'" I would chant. "Three singing pigs say, 'La la la.'" When all the animals had had their say, I would turn hopefully to J.P. on the book's last line, an unintentionally poignant question: "(It's quiet now. What do *you* say?)." I never got an answer.

J.P. loved the sounds of individual words so much that when one struck his fancy he would laugh out loud and make us repeat it dozens of times. Vocabulary was always his strength, as later we would discover is typical of kids with fragile X. Words stick out like trapunto in a J.P. sentence: when J.P. was eight or nine his otherwise garbled sentences were studded with knock-'em-dead words—*glamorous* and *sheepish*, *nauseous* and *ravishing*. His vocabulary is probably more sophisticated than those of many of his fragile X cohort; after all, he inherited other genes than the blasted FMR1 gene, and his mother is an avid reader and writer. As a child, I loved to flip through the dictionary and discover new words. I spent one summer showing off my mastery of the supposedly longest word in the English language, *antidisestablishmentarianism*, spelling it aloud as fast as I could to all who would listen. Every cent of the first money I ever received as a gift—the fives and tens tucked into cards at my First Communion—I spent on books: brightly colored hardback versions of the Bobbsey Twins and Nancy Drew.

Today, at age twenty-one, J.P. reads at about the third-grade level, and then only when highly motivated. Books are too complex to hold his attention, but he easily reads items in *People* or *Country Weekly*, a country-music magazine that he discovered on a visit to Florida and now receives by subscription. He loves newspapers, especially the racing section of the sports page, the TV listings, and the headlines of our city's daily tabloid, the *Boston Herald*, which he circles as they strike his fancy. Paging through the paper later on, I glimpse his mind at work in his excited yellow circles: "Teacher Caught in Sex Romp with Student" or "Moose Loose in Beantown."

As with other children with fragile X, J.P.'s academic skills were more impressive in his early years than in puberty, when the cognitive gap widened to a chasm. At age six, J.P. recognized so many words by sight that even his classmates were impressed. Years later, when a new student to J.P.'s fifth-grade class taunted J.P., the teachers called a class meeting and asked his classmates to explain to the new boy how J.P. was different. With remarkable accuracy and matter-of-factness, his classmates enumerated J.P.'s differences: that it was hard for J.P. to sit still, and that math was difficult, but, as they recalled it (how I cherish this memory!), he had been one of the few kids able to read in kindergarten.

MY OWN LIFE as a reader began in first grade at St. Peter's School in Cambridge, Massachusetts, where in September 1960 my family—my parents, my brother, Mark, and I—moved for the school year while my father got a master's degree in law at Harvard. The world opened up for me that year: meaning burst out at me from words on the page, and time took shape in the hands of my Alice in Wonderland wristwatch. My after-school playmate was a *boy*, for heaven's sake, the only kid my age in the apartment building. I could take nothing for granted in this new life, not even the girl I thought I was in St. Louis.

I'm sure my parents have less magical memories of that year. Ensconced in a dark apartment in Cambridge, a city part Old World ivy and Kennedy glamour, part rude Easterners and iron piles of dirty snow, the four of us were in terra incognita. My parents had no advantage over me here, for we all faced our own unique challenges. My father, a law professor, had to face the challenge of being a student again at thirty-three, not to mention Harvard snobbery. My mother was expecting her third child after having lost two babies, and was so plagued by morning sickness that, with the perverse taste buds of pregnancy, she could only keep down canned SpaghettiOs. In February, she gave birth to my sister Cathy, who had a host of medical problems. My brother, a mere four-year-old baby in my eyes, didn't yet attend school, so that left me with a world to conquer and no one paying close attention.

I made a place for myself in a crowded class of fifty first-graders, becoming something of a teacher's pet. My parents were now no longer the only important voices in my life, though I never forgot my roots. One day it was my turn to read aloud in class.

"She laughed and laughed and laughed," I read in my flat midwestern accent. Sister Mary Stephen stopped me right there.

"No, Clare," she said, "she lahfed and lahfed and lahfed." Her broad *a* was as astonishing to me as if she spoke in tongues.

"No," I said primly, "that's not how *we* say it." Usually respectful of authority, I would not capitulate on a matter so intimate as language. I asserted my origins in the face of cultural tyranny. Sister tried again, but I would not budge. Later she told my parents the story and they all had a "lahf" at my expense.

J.P.'S SPEECH, so late in developing, is as hard for strangers to understand as the broad Boston accent was for me as a child. It is rapid and has an odd rhythm that is a function of both unusual syntax and intonation. Speech therapists call this cluttered speech. As a mother, I feel I am always filling in the blanks, creating the text like some literal embodiment of the reader imagined by literary critic Stanley Fish, asking my son to repeat himself over and over and still finally concluding that the "text in the room" is my own. In fact, we are cocreators, he and I, and when meaning leaps out in our midst we grab it by either side, like a trophy with two handles.

But it is not just how he says it, but what he says, that turns J.P.'s speech into riddle. Children with fragile X find it difficult to answer a direct question and offer answers that are oblique at best. Although this is an issue of cognitive processing, their nervous systems also cannot withstand a direct approach, and they often cannot make eye contact with their questioner. Teachers of those with fragile X are encouraged to sit side by side with their student, so that the child can take in the information without having to fend off the barrage of sensations a direct gaze can unleash. Eye contact is one of the behaviors our culture demands, especially in children—"Look me in the eye when you talk to me!"—and family and teachers alike have had to learn that J.P. is not being disrespectful or inattentive when he turns aside, but shielding himself from an unbearable intimacy.

Sidelong when I crave head-on, oblique when I yearn for a direct embrace—the posture I take in communicating with my son goes against the grain of a mother's instinct. But in some sense it is really where all of us are situated: mothers and children, husbands and wives, lovers, friends—maneuvering carefully in the narrow gap between intimacy and isolation. J.P.'s and my movements are just a little more stylized, like Noh theater when those around us seem to be acting in a Broadway play; while they are bursting into song, declaiming unself-consciously their well-scripted dialogue, my son and I are moving stiffly in our elaborate costumes, acting out a scenario half signed, half spoken. Context is all.

One morning when he was ten years old, J.P. was eating breakfast and announced, "You're a great cook, Mommy." Since he was eating peach yogurt from a carton and store-bought muffins, this compliment was a stretch. A minute or two later, he stood up, juice glass in hand, and said, "This juice is delicious. It tastes like popcorn-marmalade." He then came over and hugged me with a twinkle in his eye that usually means he's been up to mischief. Suddenly, his meaning dawned. The night before, I had microwaved popcorn and put the uneaten portion in a bag that I left on top of the breadbox.

"Did you eat the popcorn in the bag?" I asked J.P.

"Yes," he answered promptly. Evidently he had found the popcorn before I got up that morning, and, in his own indirect way, wanted to fess up to finishing it. Orange juice plus popcorn equals popcorn-marmalade. The metaphor is decoded.

Metaphor is J.P.'s forte. The moon is a cinnamon cookie, J.P. declared one crisp autumn night at age eight. The summer he attended a special school for children more severely affected by their disabilities than he is, he struggled with his self-image and seemed anguished that his parents thought he belonged there.

The other kids, he wailed, were "diaper-wipes"! Recently, when I asked why he had put mayonnaise on his peanut butter sandwich, he answered happily, "See, it looks like snow!"

When assigned to write poems in elementary school, J.P. often came up with striking images that once earned him the chance to have his poem read at a school assembly. Asked to describe his concept of "wilderness" in terms of the five senses, J.P. began:

> *Wilderness feels like*
> *a rainy day*
> *soft as a mealworm*
> *safe from cars.*
>
> *Wilderness tastes like*
> *apples and*
> *cockroaches.*

J.P. has a way of capturing the essence of people he knows with the names he devises for them, either compounds of his own invention or the names of characters from fairy tales, Disney, or TV. You could know something quite accurate about each of the female classmates he describes in this excerpt from his eighth-grade classroom journal. Asked to reflect on what distracts him in school, he dictated this to his teacher:

> Sometimes I think about girlfriends too much. I think about their pigtails and their loveliness. I daydream about Heather, who looks like a mermaid, and Jessie, who looks like Snow White, Melissa, who looks like Tinker Bell, and Shannon who reminds me of her beautiness, and Liana who reminds me of Minnie Mouse, and Danielle who reminds me of Barbie. All these ladies make my mind run like the *Titanic*. I need to kick them out of my skull so I can slow down and learn.

J.P. makes lightning-fast associations and then acts on them. One night recently, J.P., a friend, and I go to J.P.'s favorite restaurant, Vinny T's, where J.P. likes to devour a basket of focaccia and a bowl of roasted garlic in olive oil. The waitress introduces herself as Joan.

"Hi, Joan," J.P. says, uncharacteristically looking right at her. "I'm your biggest fan." She laughs and goes to get our drink orders. I find this odd, but then, I'm used to odd. Now J.P. puts his cloth napkin over his head and says to the two of us in a fake accent, "I'm from Frahnce." This is just as puzzling.

Then Joan returns with the drinks, and J.P. says quickly, "Thanks, Joan of Arc." My friend and I finally get it and burst out laughing. Poor Joan may still be trying to figure us out.

WHEN MY FAMILY left Cambridge for St. Louis at the end of the school year, Sister Mary Stephen presented me with a statue of the Infant of Prague, a representation of the Baby Jesus complete with a jeweled tiara that, when not on the infant's dented skull, resided in a clear plastic box. The nuns had sewn for the statue a pink brocade robe and pink satin cape, trimmed in gold rickrack and lace; the cape really tied, which thrilled me because the clothes were removable, like doll's clothes. I liked the idea that you could deck out the infant and make him into a royal king and then, in a couple of steps, make him an undistinguished baby again.

The other gift I received when I left Cambridge was just as wonderful, just as premonitory. I had made a friend during this momentous year in a little girl with large round eyes and long black braids. It was my friend Kathleen who gave me my first copy of my favorite book in the world, *Alice in Wonderland*. A book and a baby, the two poles of my future, defined Boston for me until I returned at twenty-one to go to graduate school in English.

Alice would become my private heroine, this curious and

gutsy but perpetually polite Victorian girl. When I was eighteen, I even got to be Alice in a production of an experimental version of *Alice in Wonderland* at my brother's Catholic boys' high school; asked why he chose me, the director said that it was pure typecasting. With my brother playing the Mad Hatter, I tumbled in somersaults through the hands of my fellow actors down the rabbit hole into a bizarre new world.

THE WORLD OF THOSE with fragile X syndrome, as for many cognitively challenged persons, is highly concrete, making abstractions like mathematics almost unconquerable. But this world yields the key to other mysteries. At Mass on Christmas Day, J.P. sees wine and bread carried to the altar in the offertory procession and exclaims, "Yuck! I hate blood!" J.P. made his First Communion, thanks to a loving and patient nun who gave him religious instruction, so he knew the Catholic belief that bread and wine are transformed into the body and blood of Christ in the sacrament of the Mass. No sooner has he said "yuck" on this Christmas morning than he announces, "I'll go to Communion," and rubs his stomach—"yum-yum!" He has an instinctive sacramental understanding of the world, which must be both terrifying and consoling. The Christmas Gospel according to John announces, "The Word became flesh and dwelt among us." I know this is true because of my son.

J.P. is utterly literal. When the priest intones the ceremonial command, "Let us stand," my son answers loudly and incredulously, "Why?" After the ritual "Alleluia," he cheers, "That's right, guys!" An old ceremony glints with new shine in my son's ebullient presence.

Our life together has a surreal extravagance. At this same Christmas Mass, J.P. enters the church, only to rush up to the crèche and dramatically kiss the statue of the Infant Jesus in the manger. He then looks up at the candelabrum on the altar and says so all can hear, "There's a menorah!" One moment he is singing with the congregation, making up some of the words of the hymn in a kind of riff on love, and the next he is crying. I cannot predict or control his moods or their expression.

J.P. speaks in shifting registers of diction that mirror the shifting tectonic plates of his emotions. One moment he drawls like a country song, "I've got my mom and that's all I need"; the next he invokes fairy tale, as he trills the *r*: "You look r-r-r-ravishing! You're the princess of my dreams." Sometimes he speaks in what I think of as his "We Are the World" mode: "We are a famil-y, living in harmon-y," he croons as I fix our dinner. Occasionally, he lapses into the language of old-fashioned storybooks, as when he intones, "Woe is me," over his cereal bowl.

Then there is the language of romance novels, often heard during middle school as he fell in love with a new classmate every week. "I'm going to make her my wife," he declared at age thirteen of his first love, Shannon, whom he also once called "my little rose blossom." Another morning he stopped eating breakfast dramatically, saying, hand on his heart: "I think I'm in love. . . . My heart is beating. . . . She's my heart, my soul, my beloved. . . . It's my destiny!" Of these love affairs, which come and go in the middle school classroom with such velocity and publicity, he dreamily remarked one day, after listing all his classmates' crushes, "Love is in the air."

J.P.'s speech depends on formulas he has picked up, with startling accuracy, from television, books, movies, and pop-culture magazines. He knows the lyrics to a staggering number of pop songs, knows Britney Spears's latest outrage, knows that a menorah is part of Chanukah, and knows the Spanish expression "*Vámanos!*" This makes him a kind of poster child for Richard Dawkins's notion of the meme, a bit of information that circulates in the cultural atmosphere and infects human minds like a virus, replicating itself like DNA. As a writing teacher and academic dean, I am a watchdog of originality, but a concept once crystal-clear has become blurred in an age of instant and osmotic communication.

When I taught at Harvard I was forced to report a student who plagiarized almost all her papers in my seminar. She called me at home at night and wailed, "How could you do this? You're a mother!" She meant to appeal to my sense of compassion, as if motherhood overrode my sense of justice, the rush of hormones flooding the cool honeycomb of my brain. I was insulted, and yet, years later, I see a deeper sense in which motherhood muddies the transparency of originality. We all owe something to those from whom we came. To be human is to set foot on Darwin's "entangled bank," a rich loam of mutual dependence and dazzling diversity. Genetically, we are all copycats of our ancestors, except those of us whose text carries mutations. In that sense, my son is a true original, and yet even his originality carries echoes of the long and resonant history of the language his species speaks.

Going to school the Friday before the New England Patriots are playing in the Super Bowl in February 2005, J.P. tells me that his teacher, whom he adores, has told them to wear their Patriots gear. "Ms. Dacey told us," he warns me, "and she's the boss." But then his face softens. "She's my woman," he says, giggling, "my honey." And then, with a wide grin, "She's as lovely as a peacock's tail." My son, in sweatpants and a Patriots T-shirt, trails the glory of the Song of Solomon.

I USED TO THINK that I was not the right mother for J.P., that a writer, a teacher of literature, a nonstop talker should not have been matched with a boy who failed to speak for so long, and who finally spoke in a way that is, by most standards, disordered in almost every respect. It has been a strenuous process to understand his needs these past twenty-one years, to hear what he was saying in his shrieks, his abortive word attempts, his single words, his rapid, cluttered speech. I have to listen carefully, to decipher what I can and infer the rest; I have to catch meaning on the fly, feint and dodge to feel it hit, but when it does... it hits home.

If I am honest, I have sometimes found a perverse pleasure in my lonely quest for meaning. Stevens's "The Motive for Meta-aphor" begins with a startling accusation or perhaps a confession:

> You like it under the trees in autumn,
> Because everything is half dead.
> The wind moves like a cripple among the leaves
> And repeats words without meaning.
>
> In the same way, you were happy in spring,
> With the half colors of quarter-things,
> The slightly brighter sky, the melting clouds,
> The single bird, the obscure moon—
>
> The obscure moon lighting an obscure world
> Of things that would never be quite expressed,
> Where you yourself were not quite yourself
> And did not want nor have to be....

Born into a family in which many things are spoken but much is unsaid, I was used to catching glimmers of the hot truth that pulsed around me and speaking of everything but. Hiding out from my own desires, afraid to test myself in the full-time academic job market, I didn't always mind the isolation that came with being the mother of a special-needs child. It gave me an excuse not to "have to be" myself.

My love for poetry, its melting obscurity, is met by the poetry of J.P.'s speech, our symbiosis as inevitable and paradoxical as the

Word and the Flesh—the delicately mutating X in me coming to flower in the full extravagance of my son's mutant X. He is the poet I'd like to be, and I am his reader.

FROM ABOUT SIXTH TO EIGHTH grade I was a member of the speech team at Our Lady of Sorrows grade school, competing in the dismally named category of Non-Original Oratory. Barely pubescent, I declaimed in one memorable speech, "*We* are the *women* of the *world.*" Punching the words and pointing my hand toward the ceiling, I went on, "If I were a *Russian* woman, under a *Russian* sky...." There my memory peters out, but I remember that the point of the talk was to praise the freedom of speech that we women enjoyed in the United States. Why didn't I write my own speeches—my teachers praised my writing—and compete in Original Oratory? Perhaps I had nothing original to say. It was easier to speak in someone else's voice, the voice of popular patriotism or religious platitude. "Laugh" or "lahf"—the first-grader knew her own voice, but the older girl was afraid to use it.

When I returned to my parish grade school after my family's year in Cambridge, I felt a little set apart by my exotic sojourn in the East. While I had been away, my classmates had made their First Communion, a Catholic milestone that apparently children in the Northeast met in second grade. Now I had to be excused from second grade to join the first-graders for instruction and rehearsals. On the other hand, I had learned cursive writing already, a year ahead of my St. Louis classmates. One day in penmanship class, we were told to practice the letter that gave us the most difficulty. After a year of writing experience, I honestly thought all my letters were up to par and then some, but I obediently chose a letter that, relatively speaking, I found awkward to execute: a capital X.

When Sister Isabel glided past my desk in her survey up and

down the aisles, she stopped. "Why, you can't practice that," she said decisively. "We haven't gotten to X yet." I was mortified at this illogical rebuke, but I didn't know how to speak up and tell her that I had already learned how to write *all* the letters of the alphabet. I merely brooded in silence and wondered why Sister didn't understand what I knew and where I'd been. Maybe my classmates hadn't gotten to X, but I sure had.

TO LIVE WITH A PERSON who does not communicate in the same way you do is to know a terrible loneliness. J.P. thrives on repetition. ("The wind moves like a cripple among the leaves / And repeats words without meaning.") Some nights, as I sit across from J.P. at the dinner table and hear the same answers to my questions as the night before, I feel trapped by the tropes of his—of our—narrow life. If I ask about his friend Shannon, I can be sure that "She's showing off *some*where" and about his teacher, that she is still a "hottie"; that *Oprah* today was about "sex and death," that Ellen was "FUN-NY," and that tomorrow he will say these things again. Every night he says, "Watch the Bear tomorrow?" and as he leaves the house for school, "Watch Raven tonight?"— two television programs that bookend his day. And yet he also says every day, each time with the urgency of a new discovery, "You're the best mom in the world" and "I love you to pieces!"

I wonder sometimes whether J.P. is as lonely as I am. He yearns for connection, but his nervous system chokes his attempts to reach out to his friends. Dozens of times I have heard him talking in the guest bedroom in the dark, but when I peek in, he is holding a dead phone to his ear.

"Shannon! How aaaare you? You little scamp!"

Pause.

"What? You're going shopping with your mom? Oh, Shannon, how woooonderful!"

Pause. He laughs.

"Well, I don't know, Shannon. Are you sure?"

And so it goes, for five or ten minutes.

"J.P.," I always ask him, "do you want me to dial Shannon's number so you can really talk to her?"

"No," he says curtly.

"Well, I bet she'd love to talk to you."

"No, I'm okay."

And he seems to be. His enthusiasm for these one-sided conversations always seems genuine, whereas a live phone connection would put him on the spot.

In his social anxiety J.P. is like those living with autism, and in fact, 15 to 33 percent of children with fragile X meet the full criteria for autism, according to the National Fragile X Foundation. To put it the other way around, several screening studies have found that 2.5 to 6 percent of boys with autism have fragile X syndrome. The effects of additional background genes may one day explain why some children have these dual diagnoses. In general, J.P. and his fellow X-men are gregarious and social creatures: even as they look away, they hang around the action. However, I have seen firsthand that fragile X and autism can look a lot alike.

J.P. and I are at our local grocery store when I spot Jim, a young man with autism who lives in our town and attends the same school program as J.P.

"Hey, J.P., isn't that Jim?" I ask him, pointing to Jim, who, having just seen us, has turned on his heel and is scurrying down the frozen-foods aisle.

"No," J.P. grunts, without even looking Jim's way.

"Jaaay Peeeee! Look *that* way. I know that's Jim, the kid from school."

"Oh, yeaaaah," he says, drawing it out as if he is just realizing, though I know he's simply trying to placate me, and he probably saw Jim before I did.

"That little scoundrel," he says with a grin.

"Why don't you go say hi to him?"

"No, I'll stay here," he says in a fast, choppy monotone.

"Come on, J.P. He's a nice kid. Don't be rude." (Why on earth do I talk like this? Why won't I ever give up?)

"No, I'm fine." At this point, Jim comes down the pasta aisle, shoots a quick glance at us, and darts off faster than a runaway cart. Clearly he is intrigued, but he doesn't want a closer encounter. At some point I see Jim's father and chat with him, laughing about our boys' mutual avoidance. J.P. scoots off to the magazine section. What if he runs into Jim? They can always look at magazines side by side, bodies twitching as their senses zing, all the while carefully ignoring each other.

Some of J.P.'s classmates are, as he reminds me solemnly, "nonverbal," but even those who are verbal, as he is, do not use words with ease or clarity. When he was in seventh grade I often asked J.P. whether he and his girlfriend du jour, Jessie, ever talked, or if he knew what kinds of things she liked, but he routinely shrugged off my question. I knew that whenever they laid eyes on each other, they made a seal-like bark that sounded like "Ork! Ork!" and I found myself badgering him: "How can you be friends if you don't talk? You say you're in love with her, but you just make sounds at her. You need to talk to her." Suddenly I heard myself and realized how untrue this was, how untrue even to my own experience. Love takes root in what we feel, not what we know; communication can take many forms other than words. What's more, every pair of lovers creates their own love talk. Orking is what lovers do.

My mother tells a story of my infancy that has always enchanted me. When my father would walk in the door from work in the evening, I would light up and cry, "Ocky-noony, Daddydoe," to which my father would never fail to answer, "Noony-noony, Clarey." As my mother saw it, our passionate attachment gave rise to a language of our own, unique and exclusive.

Lately, when I come home from work, J.P. comes to the door between the house and garage and calls out, "Who's there?"

I answer, "Mommy."

"Mommy who?" he replies. "The girl of my dreams? The one I love?" Tired and weighed down by briefcase and purse, I smile and wearily answer, "Yes," and he lets me in.

One night he won't open the door. "What's the password?" he asks.

Without thinking I answer, "Love."

"You're ab-so-lutely right!" he cries.

"WO-O-O-OF! WOOF! WOOF!" J.P. is barking like a dog again, a trick he picked up from an eighth-grade classmate who has Williams syndrome, another genetic condition that confers unusual skills of verbal imitation. The two of them, J.P. and Charles, bark back and forth the livelong day, much to their teachers' consternation. This particular morning, no sooner has J.P. finished barking but he calls out, apropos of what, I have no idea, "Mom, that's hooligan-ish!" A minute later, "I'm feeling lemur-ish!" My head spins with his jabberwocky—I'm Alice in my own Wonderland, a place that is alarmingly foreign but somehow as familiar as home.

Around this time, I begin a new romantic relationship. One night I do what I have never done since my divorce: I arrange for J.P., who spends most weekends with his father, to spend an evening with my new boyfriend and me. Not just a quick introduction, but dinner and, of all things, decorating the Christmas tree.

My gamble pays off. The evening has a surreal magic that I've come to know as my version of motherhood, maybe my version of love. The three of us dance and sing and laugh and even have what

J.P. calls a group hug. But the real miracle occurs as I am putting J.P. to bed and tell him to call good night to Stephen, who is in another room. J.P. instead lets out a bark, and, without skipping a beat, from the living room Stephen barks back. My son's face breaks open in a grin. I know right then that we are understood.

# SEVEN

# Repeats

## *Obsessions*

Trinucleotide, or triplet, repeats consist of 3 nucleotides
consecutively repeated (e.g., CAG CAG CAG CAG)
within a region of DNA.... Some do change in length
when passed on, and when that occurs, the gene is often
disrupted. This mutational type, first discovered in 1991,
was termed a dynamic or expansion mutation.

—Russell L. Margolis, "Genetics of Childhood
Disorders," *Journal of the American Academy
of Child and Adolescent Psychiatry*

So be beginning, be beginning to despair.
O there's none; no no no there's none:
Be beginning to despair, to despair,
Despair, despair, despair, despair.

—Gerard Manley Hopkins,
"The Leaden Echo and the Golden Echo"

Maybe the hiccups could have tipped me off. While I was pregnant I would frequently feel the baby hiccupping inside me, and
the feeling was hilarious—almost as if I were hiccupping myself.
In the later months, I would look down at my belly and actually
see my skin twitch with each tiny convulsion.

It's funny how the phenotype of fragile X mirrors the geno-type. The very essence of the syndrome lies in repetition run amok. The typical person has about thirty repeats of a section of DNA on the FMR1 gene that reads CGG—that is, CGGCG-GCGGCGG thirty times. This happy person then passes on the same number of repeats to his or her offspring in what is known as a stable version of the gene. But some individuals are in what is known as a gray zone, a place of instability, and carry forty-five to fifty-five repeats, making them more likely to have children who have an even higher number of repeats. These unlucky children have fifty-five to two hundred repeats and carry the premutation of the gene; genetically more unstable still, they have a high risk of passing on a full mutation to their children, more than two hundred repeats and up to several thousand.

Aesthetically, repetition is pleasing. It makes possible poetry and song with their rhymes, meter, stanzas, and refrains; it marks the most memorable oratory in the shape of anaphora. But when does repetition cease to please and start to annoy? When does a chime become a hammer? Any parent knows how much children like repetition, the bedtime story told every night, the knock-knock joke repeated over and over after it has gotten a laugh. Repetition means safety, ritual, familiarity. It can also mean boredom.

*Pete and Repeat were walking down the street. Pete fell down. Who was left?*

*Repeat.*

*Pete and Repeat were walking down the street. Pete fell down. Who was left?*

*Repeat.*

*Pete and Repeat. . . .*

Repetition as pathology is a very different matter. In language it is known as perseveration; in actions, stereotypy; in thoughts, obsession. Those hiccups were benign, but some of J.P.'s later repetitions were far from benign. To look at a list of fragile X behaviors is to see the prefix *hyper-* attached to many otherwise neutral words: *hyperactivity, hypersensitivity, hypervigilance, hyperarousal. Hyper-,* meaning "over, above, beyond"—reactions out of proportion to the stimulus. In fragile X, there is too much: too much of a stretch of DNA, too much sensitivity to the world, too much activity, too much fear, the body surging with too much adrenaline. It is a mutation of excess, leading to behaviors that go beyond what society finds acceptable. Like Mardi Gras all year long—wild dancing and flung beads, sudden nudity and acts of deviance—the life of a family with a child with fragile X (or, heaven help us, two or three children with FX) is a site of public gawking and extreme exhaustion. It is more than you bargained for.

LET'S START WITH HYPERACTIVITY, an overused term since sometime in the 1980s, with seemingly every other child, especially boys, now being labeled in this way. With only slight exaggeration, when J.P. was young I thought the word had been invented for him. From the time J.P. could walk (late, at nineteen months), he was in constant movement. The first reports from his Early Intervention Program rang changes on this theme.

"He is often in constant motion within the room"; his teachers note a "lack of purposeful movement . . . demonstrated by his running ability which he does well but does so when agitated or excited, not when encouraged by other children or in the context of a game.

"J.P. will work at tabletop activities for three minutes with constant prompts. . . . The only activities he will pursue longer are those of a non-adaptive, repetitive, and perseverative nature, e.g., toy dashboard with horn, flashing lights and squeals." (Life in our household in those days was noisy.)

"With regard to sensory integration, J.P. has demonstrated difficulties with this area during class by his excessive desire for vestibular stimulation (swinging) and his continual movement even during tabletop activities."

The occupational therapist suggested we try some techniques called joint compression and brushing: lay the child on the floor (flailing and giddy as usual) and methodically push his forearms into the elbow joint, then push his lower legs into the knee socket. Using a soft therapeutic brush that looks like a lint cleaner, brush the child's arms and legs vigorously as he giggles and writhes. Repeat six to seven times a day. After three weeks of this routine, J.P. was no less hyperactive than he had ever been.

J.P., like most children with fragile X syndrome (and those with autism), has problems with sensory processing. Many of his dysfunctional behaviors are the result of his hypersensitivity to certain sights, sounds, touches, tastes, and smells. When the outside world overwhelms him, he turns to self-stimulation, repetitive behaviors that soothe and ground him. FX kids are known for flapping their hands not just at moments of excitement, but whenever the world around them is too much. J.P. also spins, a successor to the swinging he enjoyed as a toddler. He turns around and around in a circle well past the point when a typical person would be reeling with dizziness, his face in a state of bliss, my domestic whirling dervish. When he stops, his eyes still spin like a cartoon character that has been hit in the head. I've learned simply to witness this ritual and not to interfere with what is as soothing to him as saying the rosary is to my mother.

Plagued with low muscle tone and faulty proprioception, the so-called sixth sense that lets a person locate his body in space, J.P. knows instinctively how to get the sensory input he needs. When he was four or five years old, he would go to the walk-in closet in our master bedroom and pile his father's clothes on top of his body. He also liked Harry to place a four-foot-long sausage-shaped pillow, a gold velour relic from the seventies, on top of his body, and playfully squash him. Only later, when we were advised to try deep pressure to calm him, did we realize that J.P. had concocted his own therapy before we could do it for him. Using an established therapy, J.P.'s preschool teacher Pat generously sewed a denim vest for him that looked like a photographer's vest except that weights instead of lenses were placed in the multiple pockets. Although it hurt me to see my four-year-old bearing an extra eight pounds on his forty-two-pound frame, J.P. didn't seem to mind wearing the vest. Some mornings, Pat told me, he would even ask to wear it, seeking the grounded feeling that it must have given his wildly flying little body.

Other repetitive movements have not been as harmless as spinning or flapping. For years J.P. has shredded paper—book pages, flyers, scrap paper, newspapers, and magazines—hiding piles of the stuff behind the basement couch and carting bags surreptitiously out to the trash can.

"Why?" I implore him over and over.

As he gets older, he replies plaintively, "My hands... my hands," and holds them up helplessly. The nervous energy pouring through his body seems to pool there, where he feels their agitation as an alien force, like two frantic squirrels digging in the leaves outside your window. There is no premeditation in his ripping—nothing but pure mechanical release.

From his infancy almost up to the present, J.P. has chewed on whatever was nearby: shirt collars and cuffs, toys, books, paper, the arms of the sofa. When he was nine years old, his chewing almost turned deadly when he chewed up a medicinal patch affixed to his back. The patch contained clonidine, a drug usually used for high blood pressure but that he takes even today to calm his overaroused system. J.P. and I were spending the Christmas holidays with my parents in St. Louis when he came upstairs from the basement where he had been watching videos. I was on the phone with a high school friend making plans for an informal re-union that night. As I talked, I idly ran my hand over my son's back and with a jolt realized that the patch was not there.

"J.P., where is your patch?" I asked urgently. He looked guilt-stricken but didn't say a word. I had a sudden inspiration. "Open your mouth," I said, and as he dutifully complied, I inserted my finger and pulled out small shreds of patch, wet and papery. He had no doubt chewed the patch as you'd chew a stick of gum while he ran and reran his favorite video.

I didn't panic, not believing this benign drug could cause any damage. My mother, however, suggested that I call the local poison control center. When I explained the situation to the operator, she said, slowly and deliberately, as if talking to a child, "Now, get your son and take him to the nearest emergency room."

"The hospital?" I said stupidly.

"Don't waste any time" came the syrupy voice. "He needs medical attention ... *now*." I bundled J.P. into his jacket and the three of us scurried into the car. I cradled J.P. in the backseat while Mom drove to the hospital. I was still not very worried, be-cause he seemed normally alert, but by the time we arrived at the emergency room he was quiet and sleepy-looking.

Nonetheless, J.P. roused himself when the nurses tried to attach him to a monitor; kicking and lunging, he fought with all the excess adrenaline that still surged in his body. Mom and I watched helplessly as J.P. eventually had to be pinned down by two large orderlies so he could be hooked up to all the equipment needed to assess his vital signs. The patch that he had chewed was relatively new and carried almost twenty-five days' worth of clonidine. Now the drug was steadily pushing his blood pressure down to dangerous levels.

"Could he die?" I asked the doctor, not for a moment believ-ing in the unthinkable.

"It's unlikely," the doctor replied carefully, "but untreated, this kind of overdose could result in death. The chief danger is that he will fall into a coma." Soon J.P. fell asleep and was moved to a hospital room where I spent the night with him, waiting and watching for his blood pressure to rise and stabilize. I sat next to his bed and later lay sleepless on a cot, the glow of the pulse-ox indicator he wore on his finger a beacon for me in the dark limbo of the night. Nurses came and went at two, at three, at four o'clock, raising the bed, checking monitors, asking my semiconscious boy to urinate in a bottle. Finally morning came, and J.P. began to wake up, crying a little and gazing wildly around the unfamiliar hospital room. I cried a little myself, in exhaustion and relief.

As the day wore on J.P. became vivacious, even giddy, thrilled to have his mom's full attention for hours. My parents and siblings visited his room, bringing a McDonald's Happy Meal. He was enjoying it all so much that I feared he would try this again someday. When he was released from the bed he lurched down the hall, still woozy with clonidine, but rattling off crazy phrases and moving nonstop. A call to his doctor back in Boston informed me that he was having a rebound effect to the overdose: once sedated to the point of unconsciousness, he was now literally bouncing off the walls of the hospital. It seemed there could be no equilibrium for my unbalanced little boy.

I, too, was on an emotional roller coaster in those days. It was only the second Christmas since my divorce had become final. With some bitterness, I tried to reach Harry back in Boston with news of J.P.'s accident. His secretary explained that Harry was on a skiing vacation with his new girlfriend, and I can't say that I didn't take some shameful pleasure in interrupting it with my news. By the time I reached him J.P. was rapidly recovering, so Harry never felt the terror I had felt the night before. As usual, his response didn't satisfy me, and I hung up the phone feeling the burden of parenthood—at least for the moment—to be entirely my own.

This was also only the second Christmas after my extended family had received the diagnosis of fragile X. I don't remember any discussion, either then or earlier, about what had befallen us: four of my parents' five children carrying the premutation, and four of their then five grandchildren cursed with full-blown fragile X. Though J.P.'s diagnosis had pulled my siblings, their children, and my parents together into a dragnet of grief, we all stepped delicately over the net when we were in one another's company. Still, I couldn't help noticing the profusion of presents my parents gave us that year. As kids we had always received heaps of presents, more than the average, but this year. . . . A washer and dryer for my youngest sister and her husband, furniture for another sister's family, suit jackets and cashmere sweaters for the brothers-in-law, rocking horses and expensive American Girl dolls—the loot kept coming. At day's end, we sat stunned among the mounds of wrapping paper, rolling in a guilty bounty, drowning in unspoken sorrow.

FROM J.P.'S LAIR in the basement of the house he and I share, the same six or eight bars of music from his favorite singer, Wynonna Judd, blast out over and over and over: "Tell me why-yi-yi-yi." It's always the first song, always the first line, no chance to progress to other notes and words. As we drive in the car and play a CD, J.P. says urgently, "Number one, number one."

"But we've heard it three times," I protest.

"Again, again," he says, as I know he will. His reiterations lead to my reiterations—futile, Pavlovian responses that belie my higher IQ. From the living room comes the sound of the scene in the movie *Home Alone* in which Kevin, played by Macaulay Culkin, looks at himself in the mirror while shaving and screams, wide-eyed as Munch's famous painting, "Ahhhhhhh." Pause. "Ahhhhhhh." Pause. "Ahhhhhhh." I learn to tune it out, but occasionally it breaks through my defenses and then—you guessed it—it's me screaming, "Ahhhhhhh! Turn that off!"

The constant replaying of one part of the tape, whether audio or video, eventually wears it out, but sometimes it doesn't last that long. Turning the tape over and over in his hands, J.P. eventually pulls the plastic ribbon out of its case. A more potent fetish is the music CD. When J.P. catches sight of one, his whole body quivers in anticipation. With the urgency of a drug addict, he rips off the impossible shrink rap faster than anyone else could, and breathes heavily over the disk. "Isn't it gorgeous?" he asks. Soon he is spinning it relentlessly and deftly in his hands like the machine the disk is meant for, his eyes mesmerized as if he were spinning himself. I think the CD would survive him if he stopped there, but inevitably, whether in five minutes or in an hour, he will bite the shining disk or break it with the very intensity of his lust.

It is like living with an alcoholic. I can't leave a CD lying around the house; I must lock it up in a box bought for that purpose. Because I sometimes forget, scores of CDs that I've had through the years are lost to me, or will skip annoyingly at just about the ninth song. (Did you ever notice that the old LPs repeated a phrase when they skipped, but scratched CDs just jump? At least I am spared more repetition.) I can't buy CDs for J.P. even though he loves music more than anything else, and it's difficult to find tapes these days. I do burn CDs for him on my computer, but these only last a day or two before he hands me a note saying, "Tell Me Why burn tonight." Since J.P. has so few interests, it saddens me to deprive him of the objects he so loves, but there is a limit to the amount of destruction that I can tolerate.

As it is, the finished basement of our house has been laid

waste by J.P.'s ripping and breaking, but also by his habit of scribbling on whatever he can reach, including the painted paneled walls. When we moved into the house, the basement was a pristine almond color, with a thick white Berber carpet, built-in bookshelves, and stereo compartments with glass doors. Now, the carpet is stained and the glass doors have broken off. The door leading to the garage proclaims "Mom," like a sailor's tattoo. The wall at the base of the stairs shouts "Roise" (J.P.'s favored spelling for Rosie O'Donnell, one of his obsessions till Oprah took her place). "Pooh" (as in "Winnie the") is inscribed on the wall over the sofa; check marks line the panels of the doors that house the electric meter; and the names or initials of J.P.'s classmates—SB, Ben, Tina—crop up at regular intervals on all the walls.

The basement has become the dark and hidden underbelly of the house, bearing the stigmata of my incapacity as a mother. I feel shame when I pass through it to the laundry room or the garage, shame when I have to let a workman into it, shame when my ex-husband sees it. When J.P. made his first inroads about nine years ago, I made a strategic decision to let his destructiveness run its course before redecorating. "Wait till you're sure he won't do it again," my mother urges whenever I'm tempted to fix the place up. J.P. is now twenty-one, and at last look, one of the graffiti betrays its recent inscription: "Tina," a girl whose name he has been writing compulsively only in the past year, when they worked together in a supervised job as part of his program. It is not yet safe to wipe out the past. It is not yet safe to pretend we are a normal family. There's no sense pretending I can control my son's compulsions.

It was always like this. The children of my friends may have enjoyed the story of Snow White, but my child, between the ages of four and six, lived, breathed, and consumed Snow White. We went through a dozen copies of the storybook as J.P. ripped them up in excitement. He manhandled the Seven Dwarfs in squeeze-toy form, mouthing them hungrily throughout the day. We played the taped story over and over and over. When J.P. was eight, it happened again with Tomie dePaola's children's book *Strega Nona,* the story of an Italian "grandmother witch" who had magic powers. J.P. injected Strega Nona into every aspect of his daily life until his doctor suggested that he might not know the difference between fantasy and reality. I never believed this, that he had a psychosis, as she put it; rather, he chose to dwell in a story that resonated for him in some vital way, to remain in its grandmotherly embrace, avoiding a world that demanded the processing of new stimuli. Strega made life a theme park. She domesticated a wild world of terrifying sensations.

Today, at twenty-one, J.P. is obsessed with Oprah Winfrey, though *obsessed* is not a word strong enough to describe his relentless discussion of her daily show, her hair ("mopsy"—he rarely approves of it), her garb on the cover of her magazine (of course he has a subscription), her sayings ("Keep it simple," he intones as he leaves the house for school). He checks her Web site each day at school to see what topics she is covering that afternoon, and then e-mails me at work: "Oprah best show." The Oprahfication of J.P.'s life is comical, annoying, banal, intriguing, and, finally, transparent. The function Oprah serves, like her sisters Snow White and Strega Nona, is to simplify J.P.'s life; her motto ironically explains why my son loves her. For his world—our world—is so decidedly *not* simple. At the physical level, it is noisy, bright, odorous, abrasive or eerily slick. You can't count on much: different people in your life make different demands on you, have different standards (Mom, Dad, teachers, bus driver, the man behind the checkout counter). The day's schedule changes, too, as people change their minds, it snows, or the car breaks down. But *Oprah* appears every day, at 4:00 p.m. on the dot, and the afternoon falls into place. There is Before *Oprah* and After *Oprah,* and in some sense they matter as much as During *Oprah,* maybe even more. For J.P. is rarely in the moment; his favorite question is "And then what?"—usually repeated, yes, repeated, after every answer you can give him. It's as if time is a yawning abyss, and what keeps him from falling in is the scaffold of schedule.

J.P. keeps—we keep—daily schedules. Here is a sample from his journal, kept in a composition notebook, one of which he goes through in about two days. Why? Because he writes things over and over.

Thursday February 5, 2004
1. Bear 6:30
2. eat food mom
3. go SHS [Stoddard High School]
4. Ms. Dacey
5. Oprah

It ends there, though on other days he will write "6:30 Mom" to note my homecoming. Bracketed by two television shows, *The Bear in the Big Blue House* and *Oprah,* and pinned on two of his favorite people in between, his teacher Ms. Dacey and his mom, the bulk of his day at SHS is not deconstructed here. The next page, however, lists the periods of the high school day:

1. Math
2. English
3. Currt E [Current Events]
4. Lunch
5. work

And so it goes, day after day. The schedule may not change much, but *it will be set down.* Intrusions like a "haircut, 5:00" are tolerated but unsettling. And God forbid *Oprah* is preempted for a national disaster or a local ceremony; the firm scaffold of the afternoon gives way, and anything can happen. And then what?

I'll tell you what. J.P. erupts in a disordered language that his father calls ragtime. He begins to call me Shannon, the name of his classmate and "girlfriend." He says he hates Chas, his classmate who rides the bus with him. He begins to rip up his latest Oprah magazine. He retreats to the basement to sing loudly and obnoxiously. He knows I'm not Shannon and he doesn't hate Chas, but at this moment his feelings are out of control and logic is set aside.

Outbursts, the psychologists call them, or meltdowns are times when sensory input or anxiety overwhelms a person with fragile X, much as they do a person with autism, and he or she erupts in behavior that releases the discomfort of feeling too much. "Down" and "out," the directions of failure and ostracism, are experiences all too common to my son and others like him— and, let it be said, of their families. Along with my intense love for J.P., I have to own up to the feelings of frustration and shame, even rage, that come with the job of being his mother.

When J.P. was younger, his outbursts were more catastrophic. He would fall to the ground, kicking and screaming, often biting his hand or biting me. Something as mundane as singing "Happy Birthday" at his birthday party might set him off: all those eyes focused on him, the loud singing, the loving energy flood him with feelings that he can't control. Thankfully, he can now request what he needs, and each year he begs us not to observe this birthday ritual: "No singing!" he warns us, and we know that means no blowing out the candles either.

When J.P. began to use language to express himself, even primitively, things improved slightly. But language can be hurled as a weapon, too, and words like *fuckface* and *asshole* sometimes made me wish for inarticulate shrieks. When J.P. was in the fifth and sixth grades, his outbursts became more frequent and more alarming. The literature I had read on fragile X had mentioned increased aggressiveness around puberty, but this is something you can't imagine when your boy is little and giggly, no matter how hyper. Even small boys with FX will hit impulsively when they are overwhelmed, but when they grow larger and testosterone floods their bodies, a violent outburst has more serious consequences. J.P. is by nature affectionate and joking, and everything he did even in this period of his life could be matched by other, more composed moments. But I can't deny that at that stage, as he lashed out at the world, I often felt a despair I had never imagined even when we received his diagnosis. At times, we both spiraled out of control.

The worst part of the day was without doubt the transitional hour in the morning between home and school. A typical day when J.P. was in middle school began like this: Long before the alarm sounds at 6:30 a.m., I awaken to the sound of J.P. screeching or shouting song lyrics on the floor below me. He has been up since 5:00 or 5:30, and the previous night's medications have worn off. He is hyper and ravenous. No warnings I have given him the day before (and the day before that) will withstand the force of his raw energy, the crossed wires of his nervous system. I cringe under the covers, dreading what I will meet downstairs. Sure enough, I find a heap of shredded papers in the front hallway, a hunk of meat loaf in the living room, smears of peanut butter on the kitchen counter. If I dared look, I would find far worse behind the couch in the basement, where J.P. is watching cartoons. But I don't go there.

I call J.P. and begin to get him dressed for school. He is eleven, but he still puts on his shirt backward and cannot button his pants. He gives me a hug, anything not to focus on the task at hand, getting dressed for school.

"That's inside out, come here," I say coaxingly. He is laughing helplessly and hysterically, falling to the ground and refusing to cooperate. He keeps laughing, and now he is repeating a word that he has heard—*halibut*—because it has struck some obscure funny bone in his body. He won't let go of it: "Halibut, halibut, halibut." He grabs the bowl of yogurt I set out and eats it hungrily, smearing some on his clean shirt. I try to remind him to show his teacher his daily notebook, as I have written her a note there. His eyes are looking at the TV and his hands are covered in yogurt.

"Come wash your hands. No, with soap. Please, dry them! No, come back. You've got to take your pills. All right. Here is your lunch money. Be careful, put it in the knapsack!"

"Halibut, halibut.... I love you, Mommy! I hate you, Mommy!"

Now we approach the front door. My stomach tenses. This has become the climax of the morning madness. J.P. must walk down the path from our house, on a slight hill, to the street where the school van is waiting. He jostles me roughly as he pushes toward the front door.

"Damn you," he shouts and then he turns around and spits on the front door.

I can't stop myself. I yell back at him, "Stop that! Get on that bus!" He runs down to the curb, past the bus, and into the street. He looks up at the house, daring me to intervene. When he sees me start out of the house in my bathrobe, he scurries to the side of the van and hops in. When the van takes off, I shiver in relief. My body only relaxes when I see it turn the corner of our street.

One of these jagged mornings, on the ride to school, J.P. threw a book the length of his van and hit the bus driver in the head. Luckily the driver wasn't hurt, nor did he lose control of the van. After this incident, though the town did not ban us from the transportation J.P. was entitled to by law, I thought that for the safety of all concerned, I should drive J.P. to school each day. Though he entered my car more readily than the bus in the mornings, he still fell to pieces when he arrived at the school. He spat on my car, screamed, "I hate you" at me, and stood stock-still on the playground, yelling insults at passing students ("asshole," "jerk," "idiot"). I watched other mothers drop off their children, give a jaunty wave, and drive off, and there I would be, trying to get my son to let go of the car door so I wouldn't run him over.

One morning when he was in sixth grade, still taking the bus, I watched J.P. gear up for the usual frenzy that preceded his entering the outside world. Suddenly, without warning, he pulled back his arm and punched me in the eye. We were about the same height and he now outweighed me. Stunned and angry, I somehow pushed him out the door and, with shouts and curses, he eventually did get on the van. I shut the front door, leaned against it, and then slid slowly down to the floor and sobbed uncontrollably. My natural instinct to survive, to fight back when attacked, banged up against a mother's instinct to withstand anything her child might do. I knew all the clinical reasons why J.P. had hit me, but I also knew, in a fierce and visceral flash, that I would not allow myself to be battered. I felt suspended in that moment between a fear that felt like anger, a rush of adrenaline that was just as strong as J.P.'s, and something just as powerful: my fierce love for my son. Though he only hit me a couple of more times, I made some calls that year to get the names of possible residential schools should I reach my limits. It felt like a backup plan that you hope never to use. I didn't know if I would be able to let him go, but I didn't know if I would be able to let him stay.

FIFTEEN YEARS BEFORE, when Harry and I had been married only a year, we decided to get a cat. I chose a kitten from an animal shelter and brought it home to our shabby apartment in Brookline. We bandied names around—Luna, Moony, Scooter (for some reason they all had a pouting, cooing sound)—but never settled on one. At night we kept the kitten in a room we called "the tundra," a former screened porch that the landlord had converted to year-round use with cheap paneling and a gold shag carpet. The wind blew around the edges of the windows in the tundra, and the New England cold penetrated its thin walls. Whether she was just uncomfortable or had been traumatized by her time in the shelter, the kitten would not use the litter box we set out. She began to urinate on the shag carpet and in other spots in the apartment; if the mother cat hadn't trained her, my own mother warned me, our kitten would never take to the box. The smell from the shag carpet became unbearable, and I knew I had to return her to the shelter. I also knew what the shelter would do with such a cat.

As I walked down Beacon Street toward the trolley, carrying a box with the kitten in my arms, I began to cry. I had taken on this responsibility and now I was reneging, sending this innocent little creature to certain death. I had never had a pet before—I didn't even have many plants—and I had been an impatient older sister. I sometimes wondered what kind of mother I would be. I felt that someone else might have been able to train the cat and make a home for her, but it seemed I was not that woman.

Not long before this episode, I had talked on the phone to a high school friend who had married some years before me and already had three children. Nancy was a lot like me: high-strung, exuberant, yet serious at heart, a good Catholic girl. She told me that one day, in a rare moment alone in the car, feeling overwhelmed with the burden of her life as a mother, she had had a sudden urge to simply keep on driving. She would move on, shaking off her three little girls like snowflakes. Of course she hadn't done it, but I sensed the despair in her voice and it haunted me in those first months of marriage. What was I capable of when it came to never-ending care?

———

*Every night, every night, night 342*
*And counting, my son asks fast*
*And sharp as I tuck him in,*
*"Anystorms? Anyblackouts?"*
*Checks on the list of fears*
*That flood his body*

*I'm the boat*
*In the rising tide*
*I'm the lighthouse*
*In the closing dark*
*Lord give me the strength*
*To rise above these seas*

*Sometimes when I'm really tired,*
*On edge, self-pitying single*
*Mother, I don't let him ask*
*(nails on a blackboard)*
*I seize the day and back out the door*
*Chanting "nostormsnoblackouts"*
*On my way*

*Nostormsnoblackouts*
*What am I promising?*
*Lightning could strike me*
*For my lies*

*But he's satisfied . . .*

*For the moment . . .*

*Until night 343. . . .*

FOR A HOMEWORK ASSIGNMENT when he was fifteen, J.P. was asked to make a list of the times when he felt brave and those when he felt afraid. The assignment was not difficult for a boy whose genetic inheritance had cursed him with an almost constant anxiety. Under the heading "Brave" he listed "having Mom around, singing, taking a deep breath, and 'emptying my cup,'" a metaphor the kids had learned in school to induce calm. Under the heading "Afraid," J.P. listed "lightning, storms, blackouts, thunder, wind, doctor visits, and the dentist." It was a major accomplishment for J.P. to be able to articulate these fears, and the list gave me a look into his world, a place of daily disasters lightened by love and trust.

If I felt weary promising night after night that there would be no blackouts, it had been even more draining to fend off J.P. as a toddler, when he could not give words to his fears. When he was six he went through a period, as many kids do, of resisting bedtime, but he seemed to get stuck in a loop that I could not break. It was the summer Harry and I separated, and J.P. and I were living alone in our sprawling house. Desperate at night for respite from my hyperactive little boy and space to give in to my grief over Harry's leaving, I would put J.P. to bed and shut his bedroom door with an almost physical urge for breathing space. He must have sensed my need, because within minutes he would be out of the room and at the door of my own bedroom, where I had taken refuge.

I would lead him back to bed. He would return. "Pleeeease go to bed," I would beg. I would lead him back. He would return. Finally, after a dozen trips back and forth, I held his door shut, almost hysterical with the need to regroup. He would scream and hold the other knob, then throw himself at the door. The return of the repressed, I called it to myself, but it was no laughing matter. At times like these, it was all I could do to restrain myself from hurting my son: I was stretched so thin myself that I did not have the resources to stay calm as I was bombarded—as he was, I guess—by that which I could not control.

WHEN I WAS A LITTLE GIRL I had a recurring nightmare, though it is better called a waking dream, never truly lived in sleep. I deliberately terrified myself by trying to imagine eternity, a concept that was a regular part of my instruction in Catholic school. Heaven was eternal, hell was eternal, and purgatory was only a way station: life after death had no end. All that I knew of life— humid summer afternoons yielding to crisp fall mornings, second grade following first, the diary page turning over to a new day— would be lost in the next life. I didn't really see myself going to hell; my sins were more venial than mortal. But I desperately did not want to go to heaven if it meant an uninflected bliss. Huddled in my bed at night, I stretched my mind to try to envision endlessness—and it balked. I repeated to myself over and over, "Day after day after day after day after day," until I couldn't take it anymore. I needed markers I needed highs and lows I needed punctuation. Sheesh; I didn't know how God did it. And that was just Time; Space, too, was endless in heaven. Infinity was just as unthinkable as eternity.

The natural horror I felt in contemplating the endless and the shapeless as a child had an uncanny resonance in the thinking of Gerard Manley Hopkins, my dissertation subject many years later. Hopkins was haunted by a Darwinian vision of man reduced to insignificance in a world rolling endlessly into eternity:

> *Manshape, that shone*
> *Sheer off, disseveral, a star, death blots black out; nor mark*
> *Is any of him at all so stark*
> *But vastness blurs and time beats level.*

Hopkins invented the notion of "inscape" out of his desire to assert the "especial" nature of an individual form, whether natural or human, the principle of its uniqueness. I share his deep-felt need to rescue life from its own amorphousness. I write about my son's behavior to catch the inscape of fragile X, to seize the singular from a mass of repetition and somehow craft a shape that is as inevitable as DNA. I want one where there is many, less where there is more, a clean line where there is a blur. I want to hear the second song on the CD, and the third, and all of them, including the last.

The story of Strega Nona, J.P.'s passing obsession as a child, reaches its climax when the witless Big Anthony, a kind of slow learner himself, is left with a magic pot that makes unlimited amounts of pasta and tries to use it without knowing the spell that makes the pot stop. Pasta is rolling down the streets of Calabria, the town is being inundated, and Big Anthony is in a panic. Pasta is the stuff of life, but you can always have too much of a good thing. Only Strega Nona has the knowledge to stop the pot's mindless flood: she returns in the nick of time, blows three kisses, and the pasta stops. A triplet of love, and everything returns to normal. Ah, if only . . .

# EIGHT

# Saltation

## *Coming Up for Air*

SALTATION n. 1. The act of leaping, jumping,
   or dancing.
2. Discontinuous movement, transition,
   or development; advancement by leaps.
3. BIOLOGY. A mutation or discontinuous
   variation.

> —*American Heritage Dictionary,*
> New College Edition

These things, these things were here and
   but the beholder
Wanting; which two when they once meet,
The heart rears wings bold and bolder
And hurls for him, O half hurls earth for
   him off under his feet.

> —Gerard Manley Hopkins,
> "Hurrahing in Harvest"

I am bobbing on a boat in the Atlantic Ocean twenty-five miles
off the coast of Boston, squinting into the blue horizon for signs
of whales. The air is fresh and cold, though it's July, and the atmosphere glitters with sun-shot spray from the waves. After J.P.

went on a whale watch with his class in middle school, he wanted to go again—you know, repetition ensures success—so I have taken him on a trip run by the New England Aquarium. Stephen is with us, the man who barked back. That evening was the beginning of an exquisite call and response that continues today.

One day when I was newly divorced, in one of many phone calls to my sister Maggi, I tearfully announced that I would probably always be alone. I could not imagine who would want to share my life, with an out-of-control son and my own volatile mix of anxiety and frustration. Maggi replied, "Look at it this way. J.P. will be the litmus test. Anyone who loves your son will be a good man." While I sensed that she was right, I usually kept my life as a mother separate from my romantic life in the years after I divorced. It was simpler that way, and the compartmentalization of selves felt familiar and safe.

Nonetheless, as a newly single woman I began to explore some of the selves that I had walled off while I was married. Only a month after Harry left, I took a photography course at the Cambridge Center for Adult Education in Harvard Square, not too many blocks from the apartment where I had lived in first grade. Though I didn't have the patience to develop my own photos, I enjoyed going to a cemetery near my house in Wellesley to photograph old gravestones, the older and mossier, the better. You could read a story in the dates of birth and death, in whether or not a husband and wife lay buried together, in the pretentiousness of a mausoleum and the modesty of a tiny stone cross. So many graves held infants or children, and their truncated life spans startled me into recalling the story I had heard of how my father and grandmother took my infant brother Gerard to the cemetery, his tiny coffin on the backseat of the family Ford.

I took some photos of J.P., too, trying to capture a portrait that would deceive the viewer (myself?) into thinking he could stay still for as long as the shutter required. I posed him in the bathroom that adjoined his bedroom, his hair damp and combed after his bath. In one photo he gazes out the window with a sweet smile, and in the other he gazes at the camera with a hint of attitude that surprises me when I look at it now; the gaze is slightly off center in the fragile X style, but in neither picture would you guess the nervous energy boiling beneath his composed black-and-white image. He looks like an unusually self-possessed seven-year-old boy.

The summer after I took the photography course I returned to the Cambridge Center to take a course called Autobiographical Writing. The writing exercises the teacher assigned—write about your childhood backyard, write about your given name—liberated me from my academic writing and made me remember that I had always wanted to be a creative writer, from the time I began a Nancy Drew–style novel as an eight-year-old to my poetry in college. Bursting with the need to have my say, I began writing poems again that summer too, overflowing with all the things I had not allowed myself to say in the past.

Then, one Sunday afternoon in the fall of 1995, two years after my divorce, I went alone to a concert of Celtic music at Boston College, where I was teaching English part-time. I had grown used to going to movies and concerts alone, though each time I did, I felt as brave as the little girl in Cambridge who marched alone to St. Peter's School in a blizzard when her parents didn't know that school was canceled. New to this kind of music, I sat in my seat in the dark theater entranced by the fiddles and bodhrans and the searing voice of the *sean-nos* singer. With a shock, I felt I had stumbled upon the sound track of my life, fretted and vibrant, melancholy and ecstatic. When I went home, I felt compelled to articulate what the concert had meant to me, and I began to write. I ended up with an essay that traveled from the concert to my childhood memories and seemed to express something essential about who I was. I gathered my courage and submitted it to *Boston College Magazine*. It was accepted, and the editor later asked if I would become a regular contributor. I began to think I had a voice worth hearing.

A SYNCHROFLASH is a mechanism in a camera that opens the shutter at the moment when the light from the flashbulb or electronic flash is brightest, like a cosmic genie of reality. An image only forms when the conditions are right. When I met Stephen at a university dinner, my light was shining again and something took. The moment was right for both of us.

My identity was being gradually reinvented after my divorce, but luckily not completely so: threads of my deepest self were woven anew in my relationship with Stephen. Soon after we began seeing each other in September of 1999, Stephen asked me to a party to celebrate the engagement of a filmmaker friend of his, Cindy Kleine, to André Gregory, the famous film and theater director and actor. I immediately told Stephen of my lifetime affection for *Alice in Wonderland* and explained that I had performed André Gregory's *Alice* at my brother's high school when I was eighteen, using the script created by the Manhattan Project under Gregory's direction.

"Too much!" Stephen said. He had no way of knowing what it meant to me to meet the creator of the contemporary Alice whom I had played in 1972, whose adventures in a darkly surreal world were tailor-made for the absurdist sensibility my friends and I were cultivating. To me, this was just one more sign of the serendipity of my new relationship. So began the reprise of my role as Alice at the age of forty-five, as the metaphors of Wonderland began to flow into my life like tea into a teacup.

That Halloween I dressed as Alice, and Stephen surprised me by transforming himself in every detail into the White Rabbit. From his towering ears (on a headdress rented for the occasion) to his whiskers, waistcoat, and padded haunches, he looked every inch the elusive creature who had led Alice down the rabbit hole. Stephen carried his grandfather's pocket watch and I a tiny, stoppered bottle of Jameson's Irish whiskey with the words "Drink Me" on it. When Stephen and I were together, time became as elastic and scarce as it was for the White Rabbit. But unlike that rabbit, my rabbit did not run away each time I saw him. Instead, he played with me with a delight in whimsy that matched my own. Stephen is a sociologist by profession and an artist by avocation, and from the beginning I noticed that he was genuinely curious about what made J.P. tick. He had insights about J.P.'s behaviors that in more than a dozen years as his mother I had never had. Most important, he had the empathy and endless patience that allowed him to accept my son and enjoy him for who he was. Just the way Stephen had met my Alice with his White Rabbit, he moved effortlessly in the surreal Wonderland J.P. sometimes created around himself.

BUT TODAY ON THE WHALE WATCH I am nervous, even with Stephen by my side. J.P. tolerated and even enjoyed the school trip, but everything about this outing is a sensory minefield for a child with fragile X. Start with the heaving movement of the boat, increase the sensory load with a loudspeaker and crowds of people, add the fearful size of a whale and its unpredictable path, and you have a recipe for an outburst, if not a meltdown. As we walk the gangplank to the ship, J.P. keeps repeating, "I'm gonna throw up. I'm gonna throw up." Though he did not get seasick on the class field trip like some of his classmates, he has latched on to the idea like a glamorous accessory. Yep, I am nervous.

The outbound trip takes at least one and a half hours, with nothing to see but green sea rushing by and a few bold and hungry gulls. At first J.P. is rooted to his seat in the indoor cabin, afraid to test his balance on the lurching ship. We eat lunch gingerly and listen to the guide tell us that the most common whales in this area are minkes and humpbacks. When the boat reaches Stellwagen Bank, a marine preserve where whale sightings are reliable, it powers down to a standstill and drifts in the now-hot sun. With a little encouragement J.P. steps through the heavy sliding doors onto the rolling deck, but he will not approach the rail.

"The whale will hit us?" he asks nervously. I promise that it will not touch the boat, though frankly I've often had the same question myself.

I have been on a whale watch at least three other times. On one of them I was lucky enough to witness the breathtaking sight of a whale breaching, a thirty-two-ton animal leaping into the sky, throwing itself clear of the water that is its natural element. Scientists don't know why whales breach; there are many theories, but the most common one is that they simply do it as a form of play. It feels good. My companion on that trip caught the breach in a perfect photo—the whale suspended in the air, drops sparkling off his huge body. J.P. has seen the photo, and now he is obsessed with seeing a breach himself.

Suddenly, the captain spots our first whale in the distance. Everyone runs to the starboard side of the boat, making it list that way.

"Whoa!" J.P. shouts. Caught up in the excitement, he moves to the rail now, repeating over and over, "See a breach? See a breach?"

I answer truthfully, "We might see a breach, but I don't know . . . maybe." Another whale is sighted on the other side of the boat, and now all the passengers go running around the deck to that side. J.P. cuts through the cabin to get from one side to the other, laughing, hooting, anxious, but also exhilarated. As time goes on he grows bolder, racing back and forth through the cabin, hanging over the rail, giddy with the swell of the waves, the fresh air, the festive energy of our fellow passengers.

"See a breach? See a breach?"

"Maybe. You never know."

J.P. and Stephen stagger like drunks as they try to walk on the rolling boat, and they giggle and high-five as the captain calls out whale after whale. The sea holds a profusion of whales out here today—a mother and her baby swimming side by side, a whale blowing its spout, another far off whose sleek black back skims the surface of the water. I begin to relax, basking in the sight of my son and the man I love gamboling as effortlessly as the whales.

Then, over the loudspeaker, the captain points out a strange phenomenon off in the distance. A whale is heaving its massive tail out of the water and banging it down again and again on the surface of the ocean: *whap, whap, whap*. We can see and hear its sweep from a half mile away. A tail breach, the captain calls it, and since another whale-watching vessel is already quite close to the whale, local regulations dictate that our boat cannot come any closer. We are all quiet, the only sounds the light slap of waves on our boat and far off the thundering slam of flukes on dense water. Every one of us feels the unmistakable touch of the uncanny.

*Whap, whap, whap, whap, whap....*

The slapping is relentless; it's hard to imagine that the animal wouldn't tire. Something uncontrollable and undeniable about this primitive behavior reverberates deep inside me. Eventually, though the whale keeps up its steady thunder, the captain starts up the motor and we speed back to Boston. It's the closest we get to a breach on this trip, and it will have to do.

J.P. is exuberant. He is proud to have passed the test of this adventure. He did not get seasick, and he conquered his fear of seeing a whale. We are shuffling along in the crowd going down the gangplank when a woman turns to me and, beaming at J.P., says with delight, "It's so great to see someone enjoying life so much!" I am caught off guard, so used am I to managing my son's odd behaviors and calming both our fears. But deep down I know how enchanting J.P.'s effervescence can be, and the older he gets, the more pleasure I feel in it. His outbursts of anxiety are offset by outpourings of pure joy, the ship Self righting itself for a moment even as it is being pulled starboard and to port.

But I know something this woman on the whale watch doesn't. I know the enormous effort it takes my son to sally forth in the world when every daily experience—the blare of horns on the road, the smell of a skunk as we drive, a too-steep staircase—insults his oversensitive sensory system and gives rise to a nameless panic. Surviving a whale watch is a real triumph for J.P. He is making a stand against the onslaught of DNA repeats in his FMR1 gene.

Not long after the whale watch, J.P. went on another school field trip, this one to downtown Boston. The trip required his special-needs class to take the subway, a new experience for J.P. Afterward, in an assignment made to order for one with fragile X, the students were asked to describe their trip by drawing on all their senses. J.P. dictated his account to his teacher, who coached him on what he remembered but did not provide the colorful imagery. What follows is my son's urban nightmare, an experience many of us have every day but that our nervous system can filter out:

I was clumsy and scared to death to ride on the train. I was dying. I was pouting, complaining and cursing with tears. The train was packed with people and I thought everyone was laughing at me. I was crushed as I squeezed on; I thought I was going to burst. There wasn't a seat to sit on and I started to cry like a baby. I wanted to die as I felt the train lunge forward. I imagined in my head there were rats all over the place. The screeching, seemingly non-stop sound of the shiny metal tracks against the cold dark metal wheels pierced my ears. The lights flashed on and off inside the car like lightning, and outside the window I couldn't see a thing. It was dark, damp, and loud as my body bumped around. A lady stepped on my foot, a frightening sound lifted up over all the moans of the subway, everyone turned their ugly sheepish faces at me as I screamed with rage and fear. I felt the weight of all the people on the train against my body. I couldn't stand it one more second. I was about to burst. Then relief, an opening, like sunshine after the storm, a woman moved out of her seat motioning for me to sit. I rushed to sit and said to her, "Scram you old ham." I nearly knocked her over as I took her seat. My body collapsed with relief.

After I sat for a while I quieted down and my heart stopped racing. I looked around and I noticed the Aquarium and the whale watch sign out the window. I saw an escalator leading up to the street. A lot of people got off the trolley and I started to feel better. I wasn't so afraid anymore. People were still standing up holding on to the handles that hung from the ceiling. I watched them. Calmly, I said to myself, like my teachers had taught me, "Empty your cup." And when I said this I felt my fear go away and I started to think more clearly. I thought, "The kids in my class aren't screaming, complaining, or pouting, they are singing and laughing. It looks like they are having a party." I'm really a party animal and I wanted to join the fun. I told my friend Charles a dog joke. I laughed. Next I leaned over and tickled Miss Heather. I laughed again. Then I stood up and walked over to Peter when the train came to a halt. The party was just starting for me and, before I knew it, I was standing, holding on to Charles, as the train left the station.

NOTHING MOVES ME MORE than J.P.'s everyday heroism, when he fights back against the current in which the fragile X gene tries to take him. He has come so far from his first years, when the world seemed to overwhelm him at every turn. Creating strategies to staunch the flood of the unknown, he writes his schedules and watches his *Oprah* and uses language to light up the dark places. Each day that goes by, J.P. takes back a little more of the world we take for granted, and though he will always face a greater challenge than most of his peers, he celebrates victory after victory. If you're dealt an unlucky genetic hand, it's what you do with your cards that counts.

When J.P. was twelve, he had to get his blood drawn to check the level of one of the medications he takes to calm his system. "No, no, I hate this, I can't," he said over and over as we approached the lab. By the time his name was called and we entered the booth where the technician waited to draw the blood, he was wrestling with me to escape. He started crying and hyperventilating as the young woman approached him; when she asked him to sit in a chair, he bared his teeth and lunged at her. I watched as my sweet boy morphed into a wild animal caught in a trap. Panicked myself now, I tried to explain to him that if he didn't sit in the chair and let the technician do her job, the burly orderly standing nearby would have to pin him down while his blood was taken.

And then a miracle happened. I saw a light in his eyes as he took in what I said, and, with a vivid sense of his brain's struggle, I witnessed his will overcome his visceral fear. My boy returned. He did what humans do: he made a choice.

Sobbing and shaking, J.P. said, "Okay, okay," and, with my heart soaring and breaking all at once, I looked on as he let the woman puncture his vein. His strong red blood surged into the glass tube, carrying the fractious DNA that made him fight but also allowed him to reason.

Yet if the insistent march of DNA repeats weighs J.P. down, it also can turn life into a parade. The flip side of J.P.'s panic and frustration is a surge of manic joy that makes him as quick to stand up and dance as to sit down and cry. *The Bear in the Big Blue*

*House,* a TV show that comes on at 6:30 a.m., features a towering bear that likes to cha-cha. When the bear begins to dance, J.P. leaps up and calls for me to join him in my bathrobe, and we shake our hips and bump them for added measure.

When I say I'm going to a conference on fragile X, he immediately asks, grinning, "Can I come? Have margaritas and lattes?" (He drinks neither.) He is, after all, a "party animal," and he duly notes every holiday marked on the calendar. "Happy Australia Day, Mom!" he shouts out in the morning on January 26. "A toast to Columbus Day!" he declares at dinner on October 12. He is the first to compliment his classmates on their accomplishments; his teacher's reports always note the contribution he makes to the morale of the class. "Come on, guys," he urges them, infecting everyone with his enthusiasm. His eyes sparkle and his grin is enormous: who could resist?

ONE OF MY FAVORITE MEMORIES of my father is set in 1961, that magical year when we lived in Cambridge. Dad and I were having a rare moment alone together, one of those times when I felt the privilege of being the firstborn. On that freezing winter day my mother, my little brother, Mark, and my newborn sister Catherine were confined indoors in our rented apartment. Dad and I had walked to church together and had stopped for a newspaper and doughnuts on our way home. The sun was blinkingly bright, and the pavement gray with old snow. Without warning, my father grabbed my hand, and before I knew it, we were running down the sidewalk as fast as we could in our heavy, bumping winter coats. The sheer uncalled-for joy of the icy air in my lungs will stay with me forever. I ran because my father ran, no questions asked. He ran because he felt the urge to, because whimsical outbursts of exuberance often guided the family trajectory.

Dad's mother, my grandmother Bumbie, got her nickname from me, the first Dunsford grandchild, because she would pop over to our house in St. Louis, a couple of blocks away from hers, and ask us kids, "Who wants to go bummin'?" Dressed in her trademark red dress, she moved faster than anybody over sixty has a right to, swinging a white patent leather bag and jiggling her car keys. When my cousin Margaret Ann got married in 1985, Bumbie, then about as old as the century, joined the single girls at the reception for the bride's toss of the bouquet. She still hoped for Husband Number Three, having buried two already. As the bouquet sailed into the crowd of twentysomethings, my grandmother vaulted into the air and seized it, catching everyone around her off guard. She held the flowers high above her silver head and whooped in victory.

A figure of exuberance in her better moments, Bumbie also was ruled by a fierce combativeness that was painful to her and her family alike. When she felt ill, she attacked her illness like an enemy. On one occasion my mother, called over to Bumbie's house because Bumbie had a headache, found my grandmother literally beating her head against the wall to try to stop the pain. My mother was aghast, but somehow I'm not. Sometimes what you feel is so overwhelming that you've got to counter sensation with more sensation. It's why J.P. bites his hand: to create a sensation he can control when he is bombarded with those he cannot. It might just be why the whale slammed his tail against the water.

When I was growing up, life in my home seemed always to be just ready to burst from under the surface. It could erupt like a volcano, spewing angry ash, or it could pop up like a jack-in-the-box, ready for play. The line between laughter and tears vibrated like a clothesline in the wind. My mother, it should be said, is even-tempered and reserved, but the rest of us were happily high-strung and a little off balance—a hint of rage beneath the funniest joke, the swift slide into sentimentality in an everyday happy moment, bathos threatening to embarrass the lot of us had not self-deprecation won the day. In short, we had Irish blood, or that's how I viewed our family's quicksilver moods. Now I wonder sometimes if the DNA wasn't so much Irish as mutant, if the peculiar flavor of my inner life was the outcome of a chemical formula that went a little heavy on the CGG repeats.

When I had to choose the subject of my doctoral dissertation, I was acutely aware that this was my first public, professional aesthetic declaration, as revealing as the choice of a spouse. Only recently have I understood how instinctive my choice was. I chose my academic partner with my heart as much as with my head. In Hopkins I found my familiar emotional rack and strain supported, as I had always known it to be, by a dazzling presence of joy—a life of sweet, sharp sorrow that I tasted in private and scarcely dared to articulate.

Sometimes Hopkins's poems take on a hysterical tone, the trembling voice of a sentimental priest (Hopkins was a Jesuit) who can barely contain his emotions. But most of the time the poet holds the line: the rollicking, firecracker, asymmetrical beauty of his art is shored up with intricate pattern and steely control. Interestingly, the critic Helen Vendler, my dissertation adviser and a friend of mine since graduate school, suggests in *The Breaking of Style: Hopkins, Heaney, Graham* that Hopkins's abrupt style, with its breathless strings of stressed syllables, represents "the impressions of a poet who receives the stimuli of daily life as a series of unforeseeable and unsettling assaults" on the senses. Citing a passage from "The Wreck of the Deutschland," Vendler comments, "After the sullen dullness of the English winter, for example, Hopkins reacted with what was almost a pathology of ecstasy to the first bright day."

"A pathology of ecstasy"—I couldn't describe my teenage journals any better unless I added, "a pathology of agony." I was a teenage Byron, self-proclaimed, and poured into the safety of writing all that I could not say in the milder discourse of a midwestern girlhood. In a spasm of acute loneliness on an August night while in college, having missed connecting with my friends and my boyfriend, I did the verbal equivalent of banging my head against the wall.

> Damn it! I feel like an overloaded circuit or a stripper listening to bumping music without an audience! Why should the fact that David is six hundred miles away keep me from seeing him at the moment I want to? Why should the fact that I may have missed a phone call by three minutes when I went for a walk tonight determine my entire evening? I despise myself for being so helpless but I despise more the fate of a humanity that has to grovel before time and space.

Emotional excess is the common territory of adolescence, but an unusual sensitivity to sensory stimuli is not. I have always been supersensitive to changes of temperature, to weather in general, and even my diary at nine regularly records weather with the earnestness of Hopkins, if not the precision. At eighteen, writing in my journal only a couple of months after I snarled at time and space, I rhapsodized over a sunset:

> Tonight the sunset was a glory. I was home alone and suddenly looked out the back window to feel a blaze of glowing pink, almost red, crushed on a smooth blue sky and the pink even trickled out in streams toward the east. I'm not sure what I meant to do, but I ran out and began walking up the alley (north) to try to see the sun better. Then I ran home and got my camera and set out west but it was already fading and the puddles in the alley weren't pink anymore but mud. Sunsets like that just suffuse me with a powerful feeling that is like a possession by color—the world is all color (and light) and I take on a new hue to myself. But it's also like being a rat in a

cage—I'm so frustrated (not melancholic, but genuinely frantic) to see such beauty around me but above me. And it fades so damn soon. But mostly I just wish I could burrow in it like soft cotton or drink its purple streaks like wine or shake out the background sky like a blue wool blanket—experience it another way than visually, I guess.

Always emotional and dramatic, I thought everyone lived a life of peaks and valleys. Once in high school I asked a friend in passing, "Don't you feel like you're always looking forward to the next high point, and the days in between are just filling the gap?" She looked at me as if she didn't have any idea what I was talking about. It was my first inkling that not everyone rode through life to the same rhythms that I did. When I went through my depression so many years later, as my marriage was ending and the full knowledge of what fragile X meant was dawning, I thought I had hit the bottom of my life. Antidepressants pulled me back up to an anchored platform, but what I found is that they did not allow me to climb to a high perch. I missed those moments when my heart soared, when the light and color of the world danced before my eyes; as soon as I felt my feet under me again, I stopped taking the pills so I could once more make those climbs.

If J.P. and I feel the light and color of life more acutely—he with more profound consequences—we also sometimes revel in the benefits. We can inflect the drumbeat of DNA that courses through us so that it yields a rhythm we can dance to. And dance we will.

I have a photo of my father that one of my sisters took when he was installed as president of the National Academy of Arbitrators in 1985. Dressed in a white shirt and tie, formal as usual, he leaps into the air and kicks his heels, his arms akimbo like a sailor's. Defying gravity, defying something nameless, he surprised everybody but me.

# NINE

# Mutants and Wild Types

## *You and Me against the World*

WILD TYPE: the typical form of an organism as it
occurs in nature, as distinguished from mutant
specimens that may result from selective breeding

—*American Heritage Dictionary,*
New College Edition

Sheer over to the other side,—for see—
The boy straggling under those mimosas, daft
With squint lanterns in his head, and it's likely
Fumbling his sex. That's why those children laughed. . . .

—Hart Crane, "The Idiot"

"Do you think I'm odd?" J.P. asks me one summer night when he
is almost ten. I thought he was asleep, but now he's come out to
the kitchen and is squatting on the floor by the back door. I am
startled by the lucidity of the question, but I know instantly why
he's asking.

Every summer I try to find J.P. some kind of structured program for kids with special needs, but it's a real struggle to establish the right peer group. One year I sent him to a summer
program for kids with ADHD, but even in this space set aside to
treat hyperactivity, J.P. stood out. The teachers there had never

seen the likes of J.P.'s split-second attention span and nonstop movement. Another year J.P. went to a local day camp for kids with developmental delays, but he hated trying to balance in a canoe and test his strength on ropes; he simply didn't have the physical strength and agility to do those things. This particular year I have sent him to a program for kids who appear far more disabled than he is because, in addition to learning difficulties, many have physical disabilities. Upon arriving, he must have observed the wheelchairs and the feeding tubes and wondered how he fits into this world. The mutation on the fragile X gene deforms selectively, torquing a child's behavior toward the far limits of hyperactivity and sending his IQ well below normal, but preserving for the most part a typical appearance. J.P. looks pretty much like any other lanky, sandy-haired ten-year-old, if you don't know that his angular jaw and slightly long face are signs of fragile X rather than, say, the imprint of some other family gene.

How do I answer my son's question? Is he odd as in "unusual, out of the ordinary, peculiar"? Definitely. Odd as in "left over, left out, or left behind"? Never, I silently promise, as his question trembles in the night air. You're as perfect as an even number, you and I divisible by two.

But all these meanings of *odd* will dominate J.P.'s life in ways that are both blessing and curse. It is foolish to deny that J.P. does not act like 99 percent of boys his age, or that he requires accommodations to get by in the world. Yet competence is a relative thing, and if J.P. can't make change for a dollar, well, he is able to swim. He needs reminders to brush his teeth, but he remembers the names of all his teachers and aides for the past twelve years. He is odd in some absolute way when compared to the norm, but he is more like the boy next door than he is like a chimpanzee.

In fact, genetically speaking, J.P. is 99.9 percent like the boy next door, and that goes for the rest of the neighbors, too. The message of DNA is that Life is one. But DNA sends another message that is not always heard by society at large: Life does not really have a capital letter. Life is not cast in one final perfect shape: mutations are the norm, not the exception. In his book *Mutants: On Genetic Variety and the Human Body,* Armand Marie Leroi explains:

> Each new embryo has about one hundred mutations that its parents did not have.... Of these hundred mutations, about four will alter the meaning of genes by changing the amino acid sequences of proteins. And of these four content-altering mutations, about three will be harmful. To be more precise, they will affect the ultimate reproductive success of the embryo, at least enough to ensure that, with time, natural selection will drive them to extinction.

Leroi notes pithily, "We are all mutants. But some of us are more mutant than others." One of my son's mutations is obvious within seconds of meeting him, but yours, coy little creatures, may never raise their heads in a lifetime of my knowing you. Yet it is only in the study of mutations that scientists home in on the norm—known to biologists as the wild type. Knowing more about J.P. is bound to lead to knowing more about that boy next door. And the chimp? Well, every human's sequence of DNA differs from a chimpanzee by only 2 percent, so we might learn more about him, too.

"Do you think I'm odd?"

In asking me that question my son is delicately probing his place in the world. Underneath the simple observation that each person is different, J.P. has come upon the bedrock fact that he can only call himself "I" because there is a "not I." J.P. is not like everyone else, and they are not like him, because each self is unique. For one moment, in this ontological insight, J.P. is like

Plato, Aristotle, Thomas Aquinas, Kant, Locke, and Descartes. He is like Hopkins when Hopkins asked, "What must it be to be someone else?"

As a species, *Homo sapiens* looks up to the angels and down to the beasts and hangs smugly suspended in the Great Chain of Being—or at least he did until Darwin came along and proposed less a chain than a rope, one knot succeeding another but connected by the sinewy fiber of what we later learned to be DNA. We are all—mutants and wild types, geniuses and idiots—more like each other than we are different.

Finding your place in the world is a delicate balancing act of aspiration and acceptance, of the dream of flying and the earthbound awakening. Sometimes identity descends on us from without as heavily as a blanket of snow and threatens to disguise the marks that distinguish us. A score below 70 on the Wechsler Adult Intelligence Scale means you're mentally retarded—a social construction, yes, but a damning one. It's as ruthless a cutoff as that count of two hundred CGG repeats on your FMR1 gene. And sometimes identity blooms from within as seductively as a flower—yes, fed by the sun and rain of a loving home, but emerging still where you least expect it. At sixteen, J.P. wrote a simple autobiography for school. Among the usual identifiers of hometown, family, and pets, he described himself: "I am a little sheepish and a little funny and a little bashful. I am loving, sexy, beautiful, nosy, stubborn and a good sport. I love to laugh and dance. I love to boogie down. I love to lounge around like a puppy."

My little puppy is more at home in the world than you would expect. The plaintive query of that summer night is not J.P.'s confident everyday voice. To know the self as an object of your own criticism, a thing to shape and mortify, is the heavy burden of the cognitively able. It is J.P.'s mother who often felt herself an odd duck as a child.

When I was not much younger than J.P. in the summer of his sudden self-consciousness, I had an identity crisis of my own. Along with one other child in my third-grade class at Our Lady of Sorrows School, I was allowed to skip fourth grade based on superlative test scores and grades. One year I was a third-grader, and the next I was a fifth-grader. The summer in between, the adults in my life provided academic support by assigning me a whole geography textbook and a few sessions of tutoring in a hot, empty classroom on the rigors of long division. But no one said a word about how it would feel to be an eight-year-old in a room of eleven-year-olds, a little girl among pubescent savages. My parents and my teachers placed me a rung higher on the grade-school hierarchy based on the precocity of my brain; the other parts of me were simply expected to scurry along behind. The memory of my fifth-grade year is purely visceral: a rising panic in the chest and a sinking nausea in the stomach. Every morning before school I would tell my mother, "My stomach hurts"—and it did. She realized that I was trying to avoid going to school, so she sent me anyway. I sat in church (daily 8:00 Mass being required of all parochial-school students in those days) and looked across the aisle at my former classmates as if they were miles away. On Fridays the Mass included Exposition of the Blessed Sacrament, and as the priest slowly passed down the aisle holding the monstrance aloft, the pungent smell of incense curled around the pews. I felt faint, sick as a foreigner in a new land who doesn't speak the language and can't stomach the exotic food. Homesick in the purest sense, I would slip out of church and go to sit in the school principal's office.

Sister Loran, a short, stocky, red-faced dynamo of a nun, knew more of the human heart than many of her sisters in that stern and blinkered era. She didn't try to force me to return and take up my new position.

"Sit down, Clare," she would invite me kindly each morning

when I appeared at her door. In her office I found an oasis where for a little while I could be known not by my grade number, but just by my name. Watching the wall clock, overhearing random bells and bits of school business as I sat in the corner, I was invisible in the generic blue and white uniform I shared with all the other girls. To all appearances, I was one of those delinquents sent to the principal's office by the powers that be, but I knew that I had sent myself. No one spoke to me; I simply sat there watching an orange goldfish swim around in a bowl. It was a good girl's time-out, a step out of time and place. By the end of Mass, my stomachache would subside and I could walk to my fifth-grade homeroom to begin the school day. Whatever had been lost in my skipping ahead—my sense of my place in the universe—was regained in that half hour of grace.

WHEN J. P. TURNED EIGHTEEN, he was given an IQ test to determine his eligibility for the services of the Department of Mental Retardation when he became an adult. Harry and I had always chosen not to learn his IQ, for we felt—and had been advised by fragile X professionals—that it would do little to reveal the peculiar mix of strengths and weaknesses that mark a person with fragile X syndrome. J.P.'s stunted attention span alone would skew the test, but we couldn't deny that for all his long-term memory and his playful vocabulary, J.P. performed many grade levels behind his years. This was one time, I joked with my friends, that a mother wanted her son to fail a test. DMR was the appropriate placement for J.P., and he needed a certain score to qualify as mentally retarded.

I spoke with the examiner ahead of time and tried to give her a sense of J.P.

"He gets very anxious," I told her, "in new situations or with unfamiliar people. But if he gets to know you, he'll give you a nickname and tease you. He's got a great sense of humor." I liked this woman from the start; she was warm and smart and I felt confident she would understand my son.

True to form, J.P. initially avoided her eyes, but a couple of hours later, he began to play.

"Who wrote *Hamlet*?" she asked.

"Oprah," he deadpanned. Then, quickly, "Shakespeare." Yet he didn't know in what direction the sun rises, she said wonderingly later. The limits of the IQ test were plain to me when I heard J.P.'s answer to the question "What is missing?" when presented with a picture of a pie with a piece of crust cut out: "A fork," he replied matter-of-factly. Despite these genius answers, J.P. easily qualified for the world the state envisioned for him.

That moment of lucidity, when J.P. tasted the apple of self-knowledge and saw himself as an outsider, did not occur very often in the years afterward. Occasionally he would call himself a dork or say he was fat or ugly, but these seemed like typical—and, for that reason, welcome—moments of adolescent angst. Usually he seemed oblivious to his differences from kids in the mainstream, so it didn't bother him that he and his classmates were not in the middle school talent show or that, on the half days when the regular high school students took exams, J.P. and his buddies cleaned up their classroom.

I guess that's why I was caught off guard when J.P. declared in his senior year in high school that he wanted to participate in graduation, to be "a graduate." Not such an unusual request, really, except that very few of his peers in the TEC Learning and Vocational Center identified enough with the high school to don a cap and gown along with the "regular" students. His vocational program for students with moderate special needs mingled only intermittently with the suburban high school that provided its classroom; the students receive certificates of completion, not diplomas, and most of them stayed there until age twenty-two, when another state agency assumes responsibility for their lives.

But J.P. was always a cheerleader for any group in which he found himself. Even though he didn't play sports, didn't belong to any clubs, didn't win awards, he asked for a high school yearbook every year and caressed the glossy pages until they tore. When the team met to create his I.E.P., or Individual Educational Plan, at the end of his sophomore year, Harry and I decided to allow J.P. to attend the meeting for the last half hour. Previously we had not included him in these meetings, reasoning that we could discuss J.P. more candidly if he wasn't in the room and mindful that he got so anxious when he was the focus of attention that he couldn't contribute much to the conversation. This time J.P. came into the room reluctantly and sat against the wall by the door, ready to bolt at any second. When his teacher asked him what goals he had for the year ahead, I waited for him to mutter, "Nothing." Instead, he astonished me by saying, in a low voice, mouth directed away from the table full of adults, "Go to the prom." He was serious.

When spring rolled around and it was clear that J.P. hadn't forgotten his wish, I asked his teacher Ms. Dacey if any of the girls in his classroom also hoped to go to the prom. J.P. had never been on a date, so we were in new territory. Jessie, a girl with mild special needs whom he had known since middle school, said she wanted to go, and suddenly I was more hopeful that the evening would be a success. Jessie was poised, sweet, and more socially proficient than J.P. and had a calming influence on him. Our next step was renting a tuxedo, quite a sartorial leap from the sweatpants J.P. begged to wear most days because, like most kids with fragile X, he hates stiff or binding clothes. He went willingly with Jaime, his stepmother, to the tuxedo store and consented to a traditional black suit and vest, a mandarin-collared white shirt with a covered button, and patent leather loafers, perfect since he couldn't tie shoelaces.

The Friday night of the prom, a chilly, overcast evening in

May, I came home early from work to help J.P. dress. I was more nervous than he was. I fumbled with his shirt buttons and finally let Stephen take over when he arrived. Cheryl, who cared for J.P. after school, came out on the patio with us to help us take some pictures. Despite the chilly air, we stood against a background of purple and white flowers and the red leaves of our Japanese maple. When Jessie arrived, dressed in a sparkly sky blue gown, her blond hair pulled back in a French braid, J.P. giggled with excitement. We took more photos, with J.P. sometimes rubbing his hands or covering his eyes, but wearing a dazzling smile in every shot.

Harry had asked Azucena, who was a nanny to his other three children, to drive J.P. and Jessie to the prom and stay on with the other chaperones. Harry's SUV served as the limo, and Azucena, wearing a cocktail dress, brought along a friend. Besides driving, Azucena could intervene if J.P. had a meltdown, because she knew and loved him. As they drove off, I stood in the driveway with Stephen and Cheryl, waving at the car. J.P.'s pride was palpable through the car window, as if he knew he'd made a touchdown against all the odds.

The car was just out of sight, when, utterly without warning, I burst into sobs. As unstoppable as a sneeze, the tears flowed while a part of me looked on and wondered at the way my heart could ambush my head. I had never expected J.P. to meet a teenage milestone like a prom, but I hadn't known it mattered. After all, I hadn't gone to my own high school prom but had spent that night brooding with my girlfriends while we sang along to Joni Mitchell's *Blue* album. "I just need to cry for a while," I gasped to Stephen, who nodded and told me to take as long as I needed.

I flashed back to the day about a year before when I had passed the driving school in my town, something I do several times a week. On this occasion, not long after J.P. had turned sixteen, I took notice of the gangly teenage boys who regularly lounged outside on the curb. Waiting for their moms to pick them up from their lessons, these boys radiated a cocky certainty that they would soon be the ones driving the family car. As surely as if one of the boys had jumped off the curb and punched me, I found myself choking up as I passed them. Every parent of a child with special needs discovers that the grief hits you like a land mine in a sunny field; it can be anywhere you step and it's right beneath the surface. Just when you thought you were admiring the green grass against a blue sky, bang, it explodes under your feet; you never saw it coming, and now you're awash in red. That's how it was on prom night, except this grief was shot through with pure joy, the sweet knowing that this moment was as normal as it gets, and the bittersweet knowing that such moments were as fragile as the wristlet corsage on Jessie's arm.

Azucena took a camera to the dance and documented the evening, so I have evidence of what I could hardly have believed otherwise. J.P. and Jessie ate a sit-down dinner with the regular kids. (The next day, still glowing, J.P. told me, "We had chicken, Mom—mmm, so delicious—and ice cream for dessert!" He made banquet fare sound like the rarest delicacies.) They slow-danced like all the other couples. (Where did he learn how to do the double-clutch?) They clapped for the band, and it wasn't even country. Okay, so they came home at eleven o'clock and J.P. instantly ran into his room and ripped off his tux. When Jessie called out incredulously, "J.P., are you really going to bed?!" he called back, "Good night, darling! I love you!" She smiled indulgently and asked for a Diet Pepsi while we waited for her dad to pick her up.

So when J.P. said he wanted to participate in graduation, I had reason to be hopeful. I figured he wanted to perform the ritual of graduation, as earlier he had performed the ritual of the prom, because it was proof that he was a man, as he had taken to calling himself. In any case, all of us who loved J.P. threw ourselves behind this new goal. In the days before graduation, J.P.'s teacher accompanied him to the class rehearsals for the ceremony, and he learned what to expect: marching in a line, filing into a row, going up to the stage to receive the diploma. I made graduation announcements for family and friends on my computer, crowned by a miniature of J.P.'s graduation photo, the best formal picture he had ever taken. He beamed straight into the camera lens, his arms crossed resolutely in the typical senior's pose.

This photo alone was a triumph that I could not take for granted. Most photos of J.P. caught him from the side as he turned from the camera, or else he bared his teeth in what he meant to be the smile we asked for. Sometimes he vogued in poses he believed to be cute, like kissing me on the cheek or putting his face next to a flower. It had been worth the price of the studio's lengthiest photo session to make this portrait a success. Luckily, the photographer was a pretty young woman not much older than J.P., and within minutes he had charmed her. "You're sexy!" he giggled, and she instantly fell for his goofy charm. He did what she asked, posing self-consciously on a stool like an archetype of the graduate, almost as if he had studied this genre and was determined to meet its specifications.

Graduation day was as wet and cold as only a New England June can be: pouring rain and fifty-degree temperatures. The ceremony was held in a tent on the grounds of J.P.'s suburban high school. My sister Maggi had flown from St. Louis to attend her godson's graduation; my parents were in poor health and could not travel to Boston. Harry and I were hosting an early dinner after the ceremony at Vinny T's, to which we had invited his teacher and his various caregivers.

When J.P., Maggi, Stephen, and I arrived at the high school field house where the kids would line up, I clutched winter gloves and an umbrella in my chilly fingers. J.P. and one other classmate were the only ones in his special-needs class undertaking this classic ritual, and I wondered how he would behave among a few hundred typical seniors. No sooner had we gotten out of the car but J.P. embraced a tall, blond girl in a cap and gown. "How a-a-are you?" he gushed, in the Hollywood style he had learned from TV. I started to relax. As soon as we got inside the chaotic space of the field house, though, J.P. seemed to tense up, until another beautiful girl came up to him and he teased her, too. When I found out she was the president of the senior class and would speak at the ceremony, I left him standing near her, feeling maybe, just maybe, he belonged with the others this day.

When I got to the door, on my way to rejoin Stephen and Maggi, I turned around for one last nervous look. J.P. was now standing alone, shorter and younger looking than the other kids, with a blank expression on his face but wearing the same cap and gown as the others, the same khaki pants and navy blue blazer underneath. Anything was possible.

Forty-five minutes later, when the seniors lined up in the rain to process into the tent, I felt a familiar despair when I saw J.P. pouting, arms crossed, off to the side of the line, with his teacher Ms. Dacey and his caregiver Cheryl earnestly trying to coax him to join in the march. Minutes passed as the kids filed in to the blare of ceremonial music, and J.P. dug in his heels outside the tent. Harry, Maggi, Stephen, and I were seated about twenty-five rows back from the stage on the right side, and J.P. was standing near the edge of the tent about ten rows ahead of us. In the end, J.P. entered the tent from the side, the fragile X way, at his own safe tangent to the swirling center. Once he slipped into his seat he was all smiles, clapping for the lucky kids who were able to give speeches, go to college, play sports; he cheered with his classmates and put his fist in the air, and flashed us the peace sign. From time to time, he turned around and gave me a heartrending grin; his joy beamed out and filled me up. I'll treasure it forever despite what happened next.

It was all going well until J.P. stood with his row to go up to the stage. He balked then, and a kind young man put his hand on J.P.'s back, trying to urge him on. From that moment, it's kind of a blur in my memory. He gets up on the stage, then turns toward the audience and begins to shout for me. I can't understand him exactly, but I think he wants me to come up. (Later, he told me he wanted me to give him a hug.) As he calls for me, the audience hushes, and I'm gesturing madly from right to left, to show him the way he has to walk to get the diploma. Over and over I point, but finally I have to stand up and shout, "Come on, J.P., you can do it, go get your certificate, shake hands and say thank you, come on, go ahead," ridiculous words, my whole body willing him across that stage. But he begins to shout to the audience, "Assholes, assholes, assholes," and then—words I couldn't hear but only found out later—"Nigger, molester," hateful words the opposite of the love he has in his heart.

Like Tourette's, fragile X sometimes makes its victim spout profanities under stress, foul words that seem to release the poison of cortisol from his overburdened system but that do not—please hear me—do not come from any part of his conscious self. They are words heard and repeated from the worst part of our culture. (Later J.P. told me he used the N-word because "Oprah did." He certainly has never heard his parents use it. It's possible he heard Oprah discuss it as a racist slur, but I think the word simply came out under stress because he sensed its ultimate shock value.)

A low murmur of disapproval rises from the students in the front. Those of us farther back in the audience cannot decipher his shouts. The woman next to me, who earlier had hushed Stephen and me as we whispered to each other, says, "He just gets overwhelmed?" and I say, "He has special needs. He has fragile X syndrome," not sure why I'm using a technical name she will not understand.

Finally, with Harry and I paralyzed in our chairs, Maggi runs up to the stage and throws her arms around J.P. The hug seems to release the spell, and J.P. allows her to escort him across the stage to get his diploma. She guides him down the steps, out of the tent, and into the cold rain, where he is crying and smiling. Our whole group runs out to him, but I'm the last. Maybe I'm still thinking he'll go back to his seat and finish the ceremony with the others, but of course it's all over. We're outside the tent, we always have been, and why did we think for a moment we could take shelter in the normal? Even before the ceremony I didn't feel like the other parents, as they chattered about graduation parties and their children's plans for next year.

I go out into the cold rain and hug him. "You proud of me? You proud of me?" he asks with red face and eyes.

"Yes, I'm proud of you. You did the best you can." I'm sobbing into his graduation robe. When I return to the tent to grab my purse and program from the seat, the woman next to me says good-bye with pity in her eyes.

By now J.P., Maggi, Cheryl, Harry, and J.P.'s half sister Lucy are far ahead in the rain, walking toward the parking lot. Stephen puts his arm around me, shielding me from the parents still in the tent watching the close of the ceremony, and I stumble along the wet grass, blinded by tears. Then I hear my name, and a colleague from Boston College whose son has also graduated runs out of the tent, embraces me, and says fiercely, "Clare, I'm so sorry. I know it's hard, but you are a good mother." She looks really stricken, as if she had just then seen with her own eyes how the other half lives.

As I walk on, an attractive African American woman, her hair in a smooth bun, comes up to me, hugs me, and says, "It's okay, it's okay," soothing phrases that wash right over me. I let myself be embraced, I let myself cry on this stranger's shoulder, I let my-self go. There is now no need to do otherwise, for I've been exposed, my son's been exposed, the day has been revealed for what it is: a hopeful fiction, a simulacrum of a rite of passage, for there is no passage from this point. J.P. will not pass on to college, to independence, but will go right back to class the next day, back to three more years of the same program in the same school, and then what? This is not a graduation, but simply our attempt to mark time like those around us. The cap and gown are a Halloween costume.

Yet somehow J.P. deletes his episode on the stage like a rejected phrase in a sentence on the screen. At the restaurant afterward, he is beaming, a bit anxious to know that I am proud of him, but mainly just solemnly basking in being a graduate, as he repeatedly calls himself. It was for him that we did this, after all, and he appears, beyond all reason, totally happy. He accepts the presents our guests have brought, he kisses me repeatedly, and during the two hours at the restaurant he never takes off his graduation gown.

During the party, from time to time J.P. murmurs, as Maggi says he also did when she led him off the stage, "a tribute to my family, I'm truly blessed." Did he hear language like this on *Oprah,* on a televised awards show, on an after-school special? He surely didn't hear it in the speeches of his high school classmates. Listening to the obligatory speeches the students had given earlier in the ceremony, Maggi and Harry and I had all been struck by the cynicism of these eighteen-year-olds. The speeches were filled with references to pop culture, and not once did the students voice any kind of sentiment that we associated with achievement or aspirations, the birthright of those completing one phase of education and proceeding to another. What they had accomplished was taken for granted, as surely as the cars they drove to school and the colleges they would now attend. The next day we read in the newspaper that a group of these seniors, including the beautiful class president, had been arrested later that night for vandalizing the high school. We laughed bitterly to think that J.P.'s outburst might be overshadowed in the next week's school gossip.

That night, after J.P. has gone to bed, I sit in my living room, washed out as an overexposed photo, and with Maggi and Stephen's help, I numbly recap the day's events. Over and over we say to ourselves, "Well, J.P. seems to have gotten from this what he wanted." That comforts me even as I feel a heavy shame, and a rage—at fragile X, at the other parents and students, at the school, especially at the school superintendent who stood there like a statue, unable to break the formality, to stop the madness by a gentle touch or just walking over with the damn diploma. No one on that stage was equal to the moment. Maybe eighteen years ago I wouldn't have been either.

I don't often give in to anger at the injustice of it all, the sheer gulf between the other kids his age and my unique and perfect son. But even as I hid my face on Stephen's shoulder as we walked out of that tent, I felt a dangerous urge to turn on the parents sitting there, so unaware of their own good luck. One word from them about what my son had done and I would make a scene to rival his. No one, no one will dare to shun my son, I snarled inside. I am a tiger with her cub, but the tiger has a mind, and at the end of this horrible day she wants more than ever before for that mind to go blank.

THE DAY I GRADUATED from high school I met my first real boyfriend. He was intellectually precocious like me, but far more sophisticated, indeed sophistical, and sexually experienced while I was a virgin. The tension between us took the form of endless teasing debates on the essential nature of the universe; he took the position that chaos ruled, while I insisted that order was at the heart of life's mystery. At sixteen I was resisting a strong attraction to Romanticism by asserting a classical belief in order.

More pragmatically, I needed to believe in order for the same reason J.P. makes schedules—to get control of my world, or at least to claim control when I couldn't feel it, and oh, boy, I couldn't feel it. It was 1971 and the world outside roiled with antiwar protest, Janis Joplin, and LSD. My moods surged along with my teenage hormones, and my parents clamped down on me for short skirts and insolent retorts. When I kissed David under a tree on a sticky St. Louis June night, I knew that I had unleashed all the chaos in the starlit sky. The slide of my pink jersey minidress on my thighs promised to bear out the domino theory in my own backyard.

"Chaos," he murmured in my damp ear.

"Order," I whispered weakly back.

But we were no ordinary teenagers struggling over sex. We were adolescent philosophers and artists, he educated by Jesuits, already writing a novel and channeling F. Scott Fitzgerald, I raised by my professor father on fierce scholastic arguments and Thomas Merton idealism, composing poems and journals that I squirreled away in my bedroom. Ideas excited David and me almost as much as the flesh. Part of my charm for him, part of what maddened him, was my almost-but-not-quite-guileless belief in absolutes. I knew there was a right way and a wrong way. I knew the rules. I played by them.

I had always played by them. A little girl who actually liked wearing white gloves and patent leather shoes to church, I had grown up to make straight As, write thank-you notes on real stationery, and never wear white after Labor Day.

But none of the rules my parents had laid down seemed relevant when I became a mother. J.P. had no clear boundaries between himself and the world: he could not—not the same as "would not"—control his impulses, and the usual "Stand still, speak up, quiet down, don't touch" were simply hoarse shouts against a roaring wind, futile and desperate. He licked my face in lieu of kisses, he put his hand down his pants if he felt like it, he spoke aloud in church, he commented loudly on people passing us on the street or their prized dogs ("Ugly little pug!"), he touched paintings in a museum, he moved ceaselessly from exhibit to exhibit at the aquarium with the attention span of the fish darting behind the glass. Raising J.P. has opened me up to the stares of strangers and a social disapproval I am not using to bearing. J.P. acts out the drama that churns inside me, and he gets away with it. He owns it. He is Puck in my own long dream, his eyes glinting with merriment and mischief as I rail against the imbroglios he has created.

And sometimes he is Caliban, an untamed savage, a mutant creature whom I do not recognize. And then I remember: I'm his mother.

IF CALIBAN LIVED in the United States today, he would be on an antipsychotic medication, perhaps augmented by a mood stabilizer and an antidepressant. We live in an age of pharmaceutical social control. When J.P. was only a month shy of his fifth birthday, his father and I succumbed to the promise that drugs could help us manage him better and, we hoped, help him to manage himself. His neurologist prescribed desipramine, one of the older tricyclic antidepressants, in the hope that it would rein in his hyperactivity and organize his thoughts. At this time J.P. was diagnosed with a language disorder and secondary attention problems, and the doctor didn't believe that classic stimulant therapy would get to the root of his hyperactivity. J.P. took desipramine on and off for four years, and we thought maybe his speech was clearer and his behavior a little less wild, but life with our son was still a struggle.

So began our long, and still ongoing, experiments in the world of chemicals. At one time or another, J.P. has been on twelve different medications, sometimes on four different drugs taken at four different times of the day. These include drugs from various classes: after the tricyclic desipramine, his doctor began trying the newer SSRIs (selective serotonin reuptake inhibitors), Prozac, Zoloft, Luvox, and the chemically unrelated antidepressants, Wellbutrin and Serzone. J.P. has also used stimulants to address his lack of attention and hyperactivity: Ritalin, Cylert, Dexedrine. Then there is the antiseizure drug Tegretol, used briefly to stabilize his moods when he was about eleven (he does not get seizures, as 20 percent of boys with fragile X do), and the atypical antipsychotic Risperdal. Each had a different characteristic effect on him, and I kept notes on what I observed in J.P. so we could decide with the doctor whether to increase the dose or end the experiment. My notes on Prozac reveal how much of a trade-off this whole enterprise really is.

On May 19, 1994, at age eight and a half, J.P. began taking Prozac. Two weeks later, on June 2, I organized my observations into three categories. In the plus column, he had increased eye contact, seemed more aware of his surroundings, was socializing in a more direct manner, and had less obsessive behavior and less whining. In the neutral column, I wrote that he had a larger appetite, focused inconsistently on his schoolwork, and was happy and affectionate, in keeping with his typically sunny disposition. But the negative column was the longest: increased hyperactivity, physicality, and impulsivity, increased aggressiveness like biting or scratching, disobedience, silliness and laughing inappropriately, poor spelling (previously one of his relative academic strengths), and trouble getting to sleep. On balance the doctor and I considered Prozac a failure and tapered him off it, only to start all over again with Zoloft.

Why did we do it? Why did we subject J.P. to the side effects that are inevitable with any drug? I cringe when I read the notes I made in September 1991 when we withdrew him (temporarily, as it turned out) from desipramine over the course of six days: Sunday night he took the last pill, Tuesday night he was up half the night, Wednesday night he slept by 10:30 p.m. and woke once during the night, and Thursday he slept by 10:00 and stayed asleep all night. But I also note that he vomited Thursday morning, was disobedient and defiant, exhibited grinding teeth, "grunts, noises and screams," and more hand-flapping than usual, and wet his pants. What kind of parent does this to her child?

Here are some answers: a desperate parent, a loving parent, a parent who believes the ends justify the means. Even to have a context for the side effects will help you understand: it was normal for J.P. to make odd noises and shrieks, to flap his hands, and to disobey because he couldn't control his impulses. An account from a notebook that I asked our longtime babysitter Kathleen to keep as we were tracking J.P.'s drug changes tells the story.

Kathleen picks up J.P. from Hardy Elementary School, and before they can get out of the building, J.P. is calling her names, along with Stephanie, his teacher's aide; he hits Kathleen, yelling, all the while trying to pick a fight with his friend Peter. J.P. begins to kick her, urging her repeatedly to "tell Mom," displaying his perverse compulsion to seek punishment when he is doing wrong. He calms down when they get home, but then at about five o'clock, as she writes in our notebook, he begins "RAGING—hitting, screaming 'I hate you' and calling me names directly with no cause or provocation. Later moving from silly (really silly: 'Penguins are taking you to the train,' ha-ha, 'the pig train') back to anger, almost rage, like quicksilver. He's getting physically stronger, which is problematic, especially when he's just as likely to grab me around the neck or leg when we're on the stairs as anywhere else."

And there you have an answer: J.P. needed, and still needs, help in controlling himself in order to function in a classroom or the community or his own home, and when he is successful at controlling himself, he is a happier person. Are his parents happier? Yes. Are his teachers and caregivers happier? Yes. But the most crucial fact is that J.P. is happier.

Still, this does not stop me from asking the question of whether J.P. ought to be made to conform to society's standards for permissible behavior, whether I am snuffing out his deviance to suit my convenience (and sanity). And am I endangering him by using these relatively new drugs, for which the long-term side effects are unknown? Since I have used some of the same drugs to treat my own depression, I am putting myself at the same risk, which is to say, I believe that for some ills the risks seem worth taking.

Who is the "real" J.P.? When he was eleven years old, just three months before Kathleen's trial by fire, Harry flew him out to Denver to see Dr. Randi Hagerman for a second time. Dr. Hagerman asked us to stop giving J.P. his Zoloft before his visit with her so that she had a clean slate from which to work, pharmaceutically speaking. J.P. flew back from Denver in Kathleen's care, as Harry had to remain in Denver on business. When I drove to the airport to pick up the two of them, I did not recognize the boy who stepped off the curb into my car. J.P. was the picture of misery: his body drooped, he could not make eye contact with me, and he refused to cooperate with anything I asked. Even his speech was a blurred version of what it had been before the trip. This was J.P. without an antidepressant. This was J.P. in the natural state.

The next day, on doctor's orders, I gave J.P. fifty milligrams of Luvox, a new SSRI. Within fifty minutes I noticed what the doctors call, with metaphorical aptness, "a lightening of affect," and J.P. smiled and laughed that night for the first time since he had come home. As relieved as I was, I still worried what such a rapid change could mean. Who was my son?

I still ask this question today. Is J.P. the anxious, perseverative, unfocused, and labile creature we see when he is unmedicated, or is he the young man who, while still showing some signs of those qualities, can introduce me to his friends and passably make his bed, who can say "I'm scared" instead of lashing out with his fist, who can shelve books in the public library at his volunteer job with only gentle reminders to stay on task—the J.P. who takes medication? How is psychoactive medication different from penicillin or insulin or cholesterol-lowering drugs? Many of us hesitate, as I did in 1994 during my own depression, to take an antidepressant because we are afraid that we will no longer be "ourselves" if we do. We are right, I believe, to take this decision seriously, to interrogate it in as many ways as we can imagine. But finally, for those of us suffering from disorders of the emotions or the mind for which there is evidence that the chemicals of the body exert an influence, the decision is a matter of seizing the chance to be *more* ourselves.

And here I see that I am back on the Platonic ground that I trod as a girl: the ideal Clare, the ideal J.P.—the perfect self who inhabits a world we can only aspire to. The wild type of evolution, the sleek and furry apex of natural selection, in whom the mottled mutation has no hold.

THE SUMMER OF 1972, at age seventeen, I had what I thought of as a nervous breakdown, though it was neither as dramatic nor as ongoing as that now dated phrase implies. My relationship with David, formed the summer before, had spiraled through that summer and into the first semester of my freshman year in college. It foundered that fall on the rocks of my innocence in a drama familiar to anyone who has experienced her first betrayal. But David had captured my imagination in a way that no one else had, and we reunited at the Christmas holidays when he returned from college out of state; even as I dated about half a dozen other men that year, I never stopped loving and hating this infuriating person who had made me Zelda to his Scott Fitzgerald. He fed my deepest romantic imagination of myself: muse to a writer, an artist herself, a figure of Isadora Duncan color flying recklessly into the night. In truth, of course, I was hobbled by a timid conventionality and tortured by a Catholic training that taught me that all that I desired would condemn me to hell.

Inevitably, I came to a crisis that was as much moral as psychological. My memory is dim on how it manifested itself; my journal is vague on its symptoms.

"I don't know quite what to write about today," reads the entry for July 1, in spindly handwriting, "the way I snapped, and what I'll do tomorrow. Shall I run away, or try to make a sensible compromise. I'm thinking I should leave school for a year (or a semester?) and dance or fly or write." I seem to remember crying and laughing uncontrollably, having trouble breathing, in what was perhaps a panic attack. My mother, desperate to assuage my agitation, took me to a local family doctor, and inexplicably, incompetently, this doctor, after examining me briefly, prescribed Mellaril, one of the first antipsychotic drugs, introduced by French researchers in 1959. This drug was developed for the treatment of disorganized and psychotic thinking, and the delusions caused by schizophrenia.

Was it psychotic to doubt your faith, to struggle with strong sexual feelings that had no sanctioned outlet in the world you knew, to yearn to create art but feel inhibited from doing so? I was a young girl, intellectually precocious but emotionally immature, who was in love with a depressed and emotionally destructive boy. I was struggling with the most basic questions of adolescence: who am I, and who will I be? What I needed was a wise and tolerant adult to listen to me, to hear my dreams and frustrations, not a chemical fix—and especially not one so powerful and dangerous. I do not remember the doctor cautioning me about side effects or even what the drug was meant to do. The only mention in my journal is to a "tranquilizer": apparently that's what I thought it was (and no doubt my parents did, too). A few days later, David and I broke up for a final time, and when another one of my boyfriends asked me out that night to an outdoor concert, "I decided to drown my woe and go—forget that bastard. Took my tranquilizer, drank wine, and smoked dope while I danced myself to a rock-and-roll trembling." So much for social control.

ONE SATURDAY IN MY KITCHEN, Stephen and I are cleaning up the lunch dishes and J.P. is sitting at the table. He is seventeen, and from time to time I try to introduce to him the idea of a more independent future. "Maybe someday you'd like to live in a house with friends," I chirp as I bend over the dishwasher. "You could cook together, go bowling, out to movies." I pause as I rinse a dish.

"Have sex?" he shoots back. Gulp.

I look helplessly at Stephen, who says mildly, "Well, maybe you would date someone . . . uh, fall in love."

One of society's most persistent fears around mentally retarded adults, especially men, is sexual promiscuity: mindless men run amok. Frankly, the same phrase conjures up spring break in Cancun. A lack of sexual inhibition is not confined to those with IQs under seventy. J.P. once turned to a young woman whom his father had hired to care for him and said, with gusto, "Your breasts are huge!" Luckily, the woman took this in the spirit in which it was said and thought it hilarious. J.P.'s socially incorrect comment is not far from the wolf whistle of construction workers at a passing woman. But the sexual dangerousness of the feeble-minded so haunted Americans in the first thirty years of the twentieth century that it resulted in one of the more extreme initiatives of the eugenics movement: sterilization of the mentally impaired and anyone deemed socially inadequate. This included, according to the Model Eugenical Sterilization Law, proposed in the United States in 1914, the "feeble-minded, insane, criminalistic, epileptic, inebriate, diseased, blind, deaf; deformed; and de-pendent," as well as "orphans, ne'er-do-wells, tramps, the home-less and paupers."

When my seventh-grade class, like so many others in the 1960s, was reading *The Miracle Worker,* I got to play the part of Helen Keller in a classroom skit. This was the young Helen, pre–Annie Sullivan, and I took the role as an opportunity to let my hair loose and writhe around on the floor in a flowing velvet dress. I groped the desks in the classroom and gobbled imaginary food. I steadfastly held my eyes on an unfocused middle ground so I didn't have to see myself reflected in the eyes of the class. But I couldn't stop my ears, and I heard one of the boys whisper, "Hey, baby, come over here!" My face grew hot, but inside I was secretly flattered. This creature was my alter ego, the girl no one had ever seen. My take on what it would be like to be blind and deaf was to be free of the constraints seen and heard every day in my parochial-school classroom. Trapped in a dark silent world, I would move as an animal, flush with the power of my own desires. I liked how it felt, my brief role as a wild child. Apparently I had already absorbed the notion that the handicapped were sexual deviants. I had also guessed a deeper secret: the freedom of the mutant.

I WAS AN ADULT and J.P.'s mother by the time I came upon an ob-scure poem by the American poet Hart Crane titled "The Idiot." Perhaps because he was a deviant himself—homosexual, alco-holic, ultimately a suicide—Crane recognized the intense revul-sion of society for those who are not normal. In this poem he portrays with grim clarity the way the typical observer projects an animal sexuality upon the disabled. If a retarded boy is in the bushes, why, he must be masturbating, "fumbling his sex," as the neighborhood children mock him with their laughter.

I can hardly read this poem without shuddering, remembering my son's mouth shouting on that high school stage, an almost silent scream that is mine as much as his.

"Sheer over to the other side," the idiot is outside the pale of the other children. But the speaker in the poem goes on to see the boy from a different perspective:

> *I hurried by. But back from the hot shore*
> *Passed him again . . . He was alone, agape;*
>
> *One hand dealt out a kite string, a tin can*
> *The other lifted, peeled end clamped to one eye.*
> *That kite aloft—you should have watched him scan*
> *Its course, though he'd clapped midnight to noon sky!*
>
> *And since, through these hot barricades of green,*
> *A Dios gracias, grac—I've heard his song*
> *Above all reason lifting, halt serene—*
> *My trespass vision shrinks to face his wrong.*

Crane's idiot is Wordworth's gentle "idiot boy" set down, a century later, in the harsh and alien landscape of the New World. Another visionary who confuses midnight and noon, Crane's boy has no doting mother to defend him as Johnny had his Betty Foy; he lies exposed to the harsh eyes of a cruel world. But ultimately the poet does what poets—and mothers—do: he sees the boy's deep perfection, the song beneath the shout.

But here's the thing. The idiot boy is still beyond the barricade: if he is no longer an animal, he is not really human either. He is a glamorous representative of the uncanny, the holy fool, an angel of grace. He will not be asked to join the other children in their play, but frightening and uplifting, he halts those who encounter him in their tracks. The idiot has no voice but shouting or singing, primitive or inspired utterances that do not differentiate the body and the soul. Whole and yet wholly fractured, the idiot is seen through the kaleidoscope of the onlooker's eye as distortedly as the noon sky through a closed can. The barricades are ours, not his; the wrong is inflicted by the gazer.

Even the loving gazer.

ON A SPRING DAY IN 2004 I have just gotten off the phone after accepting an offer to speak at a conference of the National Fragile X Foundation. J.P. is in the next room, and I know he has overheard my conversation. I want to see what he thinks about this. The words *fragile X* always make him cringe, but for the past few years I've been consciously using them, trying to put a name to who others think he is and also to understand who *J.P.* thinks he is. It's a conundrum: he didn't identify with the kids in wheelchairs in that summer program, but he doesn't seem to notice that other eighteen-year-olds don't sleep with Winnie the Pooh or ask their mothers how to put their snow boots on the right feet.

I walk into the living room where J.P. is watching cartoons on TV. "I was just on the phone with a man from the National Fragile X Foundation," I say cheerily. "I'm going to talk about you and my book at a meeting about fragile X syndrome." Instantly, he shudders.

"What's wrong?" I ask. "How does that make you feel?"

"Scared," he says. "Nervous."

"But, J.P.," I say tentatively, "you know we've talked about some of your differences from other kids your age. Do you feel different from the regular high school students?"

"No," he says matter-of-factly.

I press on. "Why are you in the TEC classroom, separate from the high school?"

"It's more cozy." He snuggles down into the sofa.

"Well, yes, but you know how maybe it's hard for you to learn some things, right? Like math or tying your shoes? Any other ways you might be different than those kids?"

"More loving," he says solemnly. "More romantic."

I'm beginning to feel like a jerk. His resistance is not just a way to survive; it's a truth bigger than both of us. But I can't help but wonder if he has any regrets about the limits that are his birthright.

"Does it ever bother you that you won't be able to drive a car or go to college like those other kids?"

"I've got you. That's all I ask."

With tears in my eyes, I finally lay it on the line. "How do you feel about fragile X?"

Beaming at me, he simply puts two thumbs up. This time, I take him at his word.

TEN

# Vectors

## *What Lies Ahead*

VECTOR: An agent, such as a virus or a small piece of DNA called a plasmid, that carries a modified or foreign gene. When used in gene therapy, a vector delivers the desired gene to a target cell.

> —Jeffre L. Witherly, Galen P. Perry, and
> Darryl L. Leja, eds., *An A to Z of DNA Science*

I exist as I am, that is enough,
If no other in the world be aware I sit content,
And if each and all be aware I sit content.

One world is aware and by far the largest to me,
and that is myself,
And whether I come to my own to-day or in ten
thousand or ten million years,
I can cheerfully take it now, or with equal cheerfulness
I can wait.

> —Walt Whitman, "Song of Myself"

"What do you want to be when you grow up?" I ask J.P. with some hesitation one day, suddenly aware of his strong jaw with its newly fledged beard. At eighteen, his once bright blond hair has dark-

ened to a sandy color, his green eyes alter subtly with the color of
his clothes, and his swimmer's shoulders are muscular. Looking
at my handsome son, I'm not so sure I want to hear the answer to
my question. In the past, J.P. has answered that he wants to be a
lawyer like his dad or a dean like his mom. Answers that other
parents might covet stab my heart with a grief that never fully
disappears. J.P.'s options for the future are limited by the genetic
mutation that colors everything in his life.

On this particular day, my son startles me with his reply to
my mundane question: "I want to be just who I am." I am used to
his gnomic pronouncements—"my Zen baby," I used to call him
when he was younger. But this time his words take my breath
away.

When J.P. says "just who I am," his face beams with a serenity that I have never felt. Growing up, I was always hard on myself, finding myself wanting in most ways. Others were more
athletic, or prettier, or shapelier, or could dance better, or they
were simply cooler. Even now I try to reshape my body at the gym,
I wear makeup, my outfits are perfectly coordinated, I don't let
you take my picture if I don't look good that day. If only I could
say, with Walt Whitman—with J.P.—"I exist as I am, that is
enough," but no, I've got to strive to be better.

When I used to wear my long hair in a ponytail, J.P. would
snatch the rubber band from it, saying, "Now you're *who you are!*"
I guess the woman he knew as Mother was the woman with long
hair; the woman with a different hairstyle was a different woman.
Did he see my essential self as a woman with her hair down, without mechanical intervention or intentional style? Since I often
wore my hair pulled back, I could not understand his insistence
that I was impersonating someone else when I did so. But I
suspect he was endorsing a kind of naturalness that Romantic
philosophers before him have embraced—and one which his

mother only honored in the abstract. Even in college, when I wore smocks from Goodwill over my blue jeans, I never failed to put on mascara before I set out to face the world.

WHEN I WAS A LITTLE GIRL I took an arcane delight in reassuring myself of my own identity, as if it could be lost amid clothes and social roles, the startling changes of growing up. With my usual fascination with the morbid, I told my parents cheerfully, "If I die in a plane crash, you can identify my body by my moles." I could recognize my own body by the perfectly symmetrical brown mole on the inner hinge of my right elbow, another mole in the exact center of my chest, and the larger mole on the back of my left shoulder. I also had a random splatter of pale freckles on my right knee just where my grandmother Bumbie had one. These marks were the guarantee of my identity; they proclaimed my uniqueness more visibly than a fingerprint.

This was long before I knew of DNA, of course, long before that invisible substance was the stuff of popular drama and newspaper accounts. As a child, my outside and my inside were totally separate realms, and I imagined my brain nestled inside my skull, like the Body of Christ inside the gold tabernacle on the altar. In the genomic concept of the self, however, my body is saturated with identity, the DNA in every cell proclaiming my name as if CGGCGGCGG sounded like *Clare*. In this telling of the story, my sequence is my self.

In one sense this genetic essentialism is accurate. A hereditary condition like fragile X is different from those congenital disabilities caused by an environmental teratogen. In the introduction to Michael Dorris's memoir *The Broken Cord*, Louise Erdrich, stepmother to Dorris's adopted child, speaks movingly of glimpsing in a particularly flattering photo of their son the "other Adam," the son they might have had if Adam didn't have fetal alcohol syndrome. The alcohol that Adam's birth mother drank while pregnant with him directly caused his cognitive and behavioral problems. This Platonic notion that a perfect self floats up there in the ether is hard to eradicate. My sister Ann and her husband James were once at a meeting with the staff at their daughter Elizabeth's school. Speaking of Elizabeth's challenges and skills, the teacher said, "I feel as if there's a charming little person in there trying to get out." To this Elizabeth's father replied, "I think she *is* out!" Elizabeth is who Elizabeth is. An ideal version of her does not exist in a faraway shadowy realm; Elizabeth is perfectly herself—just like her cousin J.P.

But today we can alter the self that we wear into the world in ways both superficial and profound, ranging from fashion to plastic surgery, from meditation to the use of antidepressants. Yet behind and underneath the malleable façade, each of us, according to psychologists, carries around a more inflexible self-concept, built up of the essential values that we attach to our identity over time; it is how we recognize ourselves, so to speak. When that self-concept is threatened, we become anxious and try to regain our equilibrium. This process is dramatic in my son's case. If I whimsically call J.P. by another name or pretend I don't know him, he becomes alarmed and insists, "I'm J.P.!" Nor does J.P. tolerate any modification of my identity. If I put on any kind of costume or mask, he cries, "Take it off! Be yourself!"

Swimming in Darwin's intellectual wake, Lewis Carroll created a world in which identity became particularly problematic: both arbitrary and constantly in flux. The creatures of Wonderland morph into other shapes and forms before Alice's wide eyes: the crying baby she rescues from the brutal Duchess is transformed into a pig as she holds it. The Cheshire Cat is a disembodied head that gradually devolves into a mere smile. Alice's own body shoots up to a giant's size and telescopes down to a few inches tall, forcing her to examine the markers of self like so many ingredients in the recipe for the "I." What makes Alice "Alice"?

"Dear, dear! How queer everything is today! And yesterday things went on just as usual. I wonder if I've changed in the night? Let me think: *was* I the same when I got up this morning? I almost think I can remember feeling a little different. But if I'm not the same, the next question is 'Who in the world am I?' Ah, *that's* the great puzzle!"

Alice looks to things like her straight hair and her performance in school to recognize herself, exactly the things I might have considered at her age:

And she began thinking over all the children she knew that were of the same age as herself, to see if she could have been changed for any of them.

"I'm sure I'm not Ada," she said, "for her hair goes in such long ringlets, and mine doesn't go in ringlets at all; and I'm sure I ca'n't be Mabel, for I know all sorts of things, and she, oh, she knows such a very little! Besides, *she's* she, and *I'm* I, and—oh dear, how puzzling it all is! . . . No, I've made up my mind about it: if I'm Mabel, I'll stay down here. It'll be no use their putting their heads down and saying, 'Come up again, dear!' I shall only look up and say 'Who am I, then? Tell me that first, and then, if I like being that person, I'll come up: if not, I'll stay down here till I'm somebody else.' "

Like Alice, I was an inveterate analyst of my own identity while growing up, never totally comfortable in my own skin. And yet when I sat on the bed in my room one day and seriously considered who else I might want to be among my classmates, I discovered a surprising fact. Though I longed for the individual parts of other kids—larger breasts or the ability to hit a volleyball in gym class—I still wanted to keep the "me" of me. There was no one whom I wanted to be in essence except myself.

AT THE PUBLIC LIBRARY AGAIN, trying to write in the after-school hours when J.P. is home with his sitter, I seek out the most isolated carrel I can find. Our town's newly renovated library is crowded on this bright March day, so I feel lucky to find a desk next to a gleaming expanse of window. As I am unpacking my things, a middle-aged man in a baseball cap shuffles into the area and mutters "hi" as he passes me, eyes unfocused. This man is familiar to me though we've never exchanged words before. He works in a local supermarket and I often see him walking around town, always carrying a plastic bag and wearing the baseball cap. He is clearly developmentally delayed. I say, "Hi," brightly, but no sooner has he passed than my mind flashes to J.P., a grown-up J.P., roaming Wellesley alone, his mom in the grave. I choke up as I contemplate the time when my son is without me. Who will love him? Who will laugh with him? Who will clean his ears and make sure his shirt is not on backward?

"Stop!" I finally have to tell myself. Who is to say this man isn't perfectly happy on this beautiful day? Maybe he's just seen his favorite librarian, he's looking forward to *Oprah* at four, and he's having dinner later on—his favorite, hamburgers—with the other men in his group home.

Ask any parent of a child with disabilities what is his or her greatest fear, and the answer is always the same: what will happen to my child when I'm gone? We try to see around the corners while we are alive, anticipating the next step to take for our kids, but around that last bend in the road lies a cliff and a windy blankness. We fear that plunge not for ourselves but for our children.

Once, just once, when I was a little girl, my mother took my brother and me to visit Mom's aunt Virginia at her turn-of-the-century house on Flora Place in south St. Louis. Virginia's husband, Art, was long dead. I remember a stained-glass window on the upstairs landing, a screened porch where a board game lay on the table—maybe checkers—but most of all, I remember the terror of meeting my mother's cousin Buddy. Buddy's brain had been deprived of oxygen at birth, when the umbilical cord had been wrapped around his neck while his twin sister edged him out in the birth canal. Buddy (his name says a lot) was probably forty years old then, a large man, even larger to a child, and he hugged me so hard I couldn't breathe. He couldn't talk to Mark and me, but he made loud happy sounds. Even then I could see the incongruity of my great-aunt, with her grandmotherly hair and body, hovering over this huge man-child. Yet I heard—or is this some yearning retrospective wish?—the hum of contented love in that house. It defied the usual vectors of time and space, in which the young eventually take care of the old and the big protect the small. The rhythm of generations was syncopated for Virginia and Buddy, but that didn't stop the music of their life.

Sometimes it feels as if J.P. and I are frozen in time. J.P. is forever a child, open and loving, naïve and guileless, even as he acquires the square shoulders and hairy legs of manhood. That makes me a young mom, still looking for child care twenty years in, performing the never-ending hands-on care that a child requires. As I drop down to the floor to cut J.P.'s toenails, I feel young and supple, but as I catch a glimpse in the bathroom mirror, I am surprised to see the subtly sagging jaw of a fifty-year-old woman. But then we're finished, I hop up, and I briskly move on.

THE SOURCE OF J.P.'S DISABILITY, the first mutation of a gene in one of his ancestors, is covered up in a premicroscopic past, in blood that was never dropped on a glass slide or whirled away into its component parts for further probing and smearing. The etiology of fragile X frustrates the family historian even if a genetic pedigree seems to point in one direction or another. It's just not possible to find the first person in my family whose DNA began to stretch. As J.P. is fond of saying, of something that has happened even just a day ago, "It's *in* the past," hand over the shoulder in a jaunty wave. Don't give it another thought.

Funny, I'm the opposite: the same words—"it's in the past"—cause me to run backward. The past is the juice of life to me. I revel in nineteenth-century poetry and culture. I treasure photos of my grandparents and great-grandparents. I still have my first dolls, my many diaries and journals, letters from boyfriends from a time when a big birthday was the twenty-first. But I'm not only nostalgic; ironically, I often am focused on what's coming next. I wish I could live in the moment more, but like J.P., my overactive imagination and anxieties make that difficult. And now that I have a child who will always be dependent on others to meet the needs of daily life, I worry about the future even more.

Where are we headed, J.P. and I? That may depend on where the scientific world is headed, those men and women who study fragile X at the level of molecule and clinical symptom. But J.P. and I have dreams of our own.

AT J.P.'S ANNUAL IEP MEETING, his teachers and therapists gather with his parents to map out the next year's educational goals. This year, J.P.'s teacher Ms. Dacey reports that she recently did a little exercise with J.P. to create what educators call a vision statement. As she begins to relate their discussion, J.P. puts his index fingers on his temples and squeezes his eyes shut. Suddenly I realize what J.P. has taken away from his little chat with his teacher.

"Oh, J.P.," I say, interrupting Ms. Dacey, "this is not *that* kind of vision."

Turning to the others sitting around the table, I explain: "What J.P. means by vision [he's still squinting madly] is the kind a character called Raven has on a TV program on the Disney Channel. She has the gift of second sight and can literally see into the future."

I suddenly hear my voice, as earnest as a teacher explaining a literary term to a class of students. *O-o-kay,* the faces around the table seem to say. *Right.* Now, back to the future.

"What do *you* want for J.P.'s future?" Ms. Dacey asks Harry and me. Just as we did last year and the year before that, we say that we'd like J.P. to learn more practical skills so he can someday live with his peers in a group home and hold an assisted job of some sort.

In my early years as a mother, I had other, more ambitious, goals. Catholics have a beautiful prayer called the Memorare—Latin for "remember"—a plea for assistance to the Virgin Mary that I have prayed every night for many years. Maybe I like it because the supplicant bases her appeal on Mary's past record of response. It goes like this:

> *Remember, O most gracious Virgin Mary,*
> *that never was it known*
> *that any one who fled to thy protection,*
> *implored thy help or sought thy intercession,*
> *was left unaided.*
>
> *Inspired with this confidence,*
> *I fly unto thee,*
> *O Virgin of virgins my Mother;*
> *to thee I come,*
> *before thee I stand,*
> *sinful and sorrowful;*

*O Mother of the Word Incarnate,*
*despise not my petitions,*
*but in thy mercy hear and answer me. Amen.*

In my childhood missal, right before the last stanza, was an instruction in brackets: *[insert petition]*. Every time I say the Memorare, I can't help seeing a soft gray stone wall covered in vines and moss, in which a chink opens. In that chink I lay my plea: at first, when J.P. was a toddler, it was "Make J.P. normal," make his differences disappear, as if his damaged system could heal up like a sore thumb. Then, when denial gave way in the face of harsh facts, it was "Make him better," a vague plea that really meant "Make him easier to handle." One day I realized the person who had to change was *I,* and a fresh slip of paper slid into the wall: "Make me a good mother to J.P." As we both age, the prayer is more specific, and maybe better directed to the Department of Mental Retardation than to Mary: "Please give him independence, a home, and a job of his own."

What does J.P. want? He would be happy, I think, to spend the rest of his days just as they are now: living with Mom, watching *Oprah,* eating nachos on Friday nights, going to the racetrack with his father on the weekend, and sleeping with Winnie the Pooh. Take yesterday, and repeat today: that's his prescription for tomorrow.

But there are glimmers of other notions. When J.P. was eleven, in fifth grade, he had to write—or, in his case, dictate to a teacher's aide—how he pictured his life twenty-four years into the future.

In twenty-four years, I'll be thirty-five. I'll be six feet tall with black hair. My eyes will still be green. I'll wear sweats and jeans and black sneakers. I'll live in the same house I live in now with my CD player. Mom, Kathleen, and our cats, Cuddles and Tigger, will live somewhere else.

Cuddles and I will be artists together. We will make collages and posters for country singers. Our office will be in my house. Tigger will be the boss, he will wear a beautiful black suit.

For fun I'll go to Strawberries and Coconuts to buy music. I'll drive in my red Honda that Mom gave me. It used to be hers.

WHEN I FINISHED COLLEGE, though I had graduated summa cum laude and Phi Beta Kappa, I had no immediate plans. I moved into a tiny efficiency apartment in the crime-ridden neighborhood around St. Louis University. All I knew for sure was that I was going to take a year off and then go to grad school to get a Ph.D. in English. I had not thought consciously beyond that. I had graduated from St. Louis U. after just three years, having learned, to my surprise, that I had enough credits to do so. Driven to cut loose from my parents (Dad's professorship gave me tuition remission) and to experience that perennial fiction, real life, I also wanted to be in sync with Harry, whom I had begun dating the summer before. A year ahead of me in school, Harry was graduating from Arizona State with a degree in political science and returning to St. Louis to work for a year before attending law school.

Ironically, the only job I could get as an English major with no work experience was back at the university, where I worked as a receptionist in the Office of Student Affairs. Not only was I working on campus, but I ended up back in the classroom as both student and teacher. To prepare to study the Romantic movement in graduate school, I signed up to study German, and I was called on by St. Louis University's English department that fall to teach two composition classes for a teaching fellow who had had a mental breakdown.

I assumed so many things about the future: that I would someday teach at a college or university, that I would marry Harry, that I would have children, that I would stay home to raise them at least for a few years. Harry made me feel safe; he was confident, forceful, and the top dog wherever he went. It didn't hurt that he was hunky and good-tempered and lots of fun. Though we enjoyed different pursuits, he sports and I museums, we came from the same neighborhood and the same network of Catholic schools. My mother had met Harry before I did, when he arrived at my family's front door asking for votes for his mother, who was running for committeewoman in our ward. Mom was so impressed that when mutual friends offered to fix up Harry and me shortly afterward, she threatened, "If *you* don't go out with him, *I* will!" Everything conspired to keep us on the track to marriage.

Harry and I applied to law school and graduate school in the same cities, and when he got into Boston College Law School and I into Boston University's graduate program in English, our course was set. While we studied hard, our grad-school years in Boston were also a last hurrah before the adult world of jobs, mortgages, and children. We spent Friday afternoons at the happy hour at the law school, Saturday nights crowding ten people into Harry's one-room basement apartment to watch *Saturday Night Live,* and Sunday evenings eating spaghetti washed down by cheap jug wine on the apartment's shag-carpeted floor. While there was always an undertow of anxiety beneath the surface of my life (my usual worrying), I essentially expected more of the same good times in the future. And why not? We were smart, educated, attractive, and untouched by tragedy. If you had asked me what I wanted from life—and nobody did—I would not have had an answer.

I simply tripped lightly along the path as it seemed to open before me.

Harry and I wed in 1979, in a large formal ceremony in St. Louis's Old Cathedral, a tiny historic church on the banks of the Mississippi under the gleaming curve of the Gateway Arch. By silent assent, we didn't try to start a family until I had almost finished my Ph.D. and Harry was working at a prominent Boston law firm. I got pregnant without too much fuss, and once again I rode the current of life. There was no going against it now.

J.P.'S BELOVED TEACHER Ms. Dacey is pregnant this year, and J.P. is consumed with the subject of babies and childbirth. He regularly reminds her that she will need to "push" and "breathe," information he must have picked up on *Oprah*. One night at home, he lies down on his back on the dining room floor and shows me how to have a baby. Straining his neck and back off the floor, he groans loudly as he imitates a push. I tell him that's just what I did when he was born. As he does whenever I mention his birth, he says knowingly, "I was yelling, 'Let me out, let me out! I can't breathe!'" Whenever I tell a story of something that happened, say, when I was a child, or when his father and I first met, he says quickly, "I was there."

"No, you weren't born yet," I explain. He cannot conceive of this time of preconception.

"No, really, I was there," he protests.

So expansive is J.P.'s notion of self, so primitive, that he will not accept that there was a time when he did not exist. And yet his imagination is so lively that he can claim to remember his time in the womb. His ego is remarkably boundless. Like the supreme self-promoter Walt Whitman, J.P. exudes a confidence in the cosmos that I need more than ever since my bloodline has been tainted by genetic mutation. In "Song of Myself," Whitman had a vision of the oneness of all selves, male and female, poor and rich, white and black, the healthy and the sick. Whitman imagined a cosmos as nurturing as a mother, as purposive as an arrow, with himself as the bull's eye.

Long I was hugg'd close—long and long.

Immense have been the preparations for me,
Faithful and friendly the arms that have help'd me.
Cycles ferried my cradle, rowing and rowing like
   cheerful boatmen,
For room to me stars kept aside in their own rings,
They sent influences to look after what was to hold me.

Before I was born out of my mother generations
   guided me,
My embryo has never been torpid, nothing could
   overlay it.

For it the nebula cohered to an orb,
The long slow strata piled to rest it on,
Vast vegetables gave it sustenance,
Monstrous sauroids transported it in their mouths
   and deposited it with care.

All forces have been steadily employ'd to complete
   and delight me,
Now on this spot I stand with my robust soul.

Such a fervent belief in teleology is hard to sustain these days. To think that there is a purpose to my life, or to yours, flies in the face of the scientific demonstration of the random chaos that seems to have brought us here. I feel that chaos more viscerally than most, the brute indifference of bases on a gene as to whether a phrase of CGGs runs on thirty times or three hundred. Though

I believe in God, I don't in my heart of hearts believe that J.P. and I were destined from the beginning of time to be the mother and son that we are. That's too easy. Instead, I like to think that we create our own identities out of the gibberish we've been given, that we decide, each and every day, to find the nonsense meaningful.

I can't live caught in the genetic net—whether it's been cast by God or chance—and accept my fate dumbly. I curse, I cry, I laugh, I bless, and the gaps in the net get bigger and my world widens. But while I hope and pray that one day J.P. and I will both escape, for now, our place is in this net. My job is to keep sifting through the patterns of shadow and light created in the crisscross of the lines, each one an X constricting and connecting like a kiss.

IN 1998 I ATTENDED my second National Fragile X Foundation conference, held that year in Asheville, North Carolina. On the conference's final day, I listened to Ted Brown, an amiable, unmistakably western man, who had grown up in Montana and gone on to get an M.D. and then a Ph.D. in biophysics, speak on "Directions for the Future." His folksy brilliance was the perfect note on which to send those of us who were parents on our way. Dr. Brown spoke hopefully of the various possibilities for treatment that were being studied, many of them in the mouse model. As he made his remarks, he had to raise his voice to compete with the stomping and off-key singing of a group of children with fragile X practicing next door for a performance at the luncheon to follow.

On the way to the airport after the luncheon, I shared a cab with a young Asian man who was a molecular biologist. He told me how moved he had been to meet real people with fragile X syndrome at the conference. Up until then he had known fragile X as a mutation in a petri dish or a mouse. He seemed slightly dazed by the experience, and as a parent, I was dumbfounded that what

I knew as beloved flesh and blood existed in the world in an eerie disembodied form. I was reminded of the disconnect between hard science and soft bodies. The young man confided in me that his wife was pregnant with their first child, and he had suddenly realized all the things that could go wrong with the fetus. I tried to reassure him that the odds were in his favor. I didn't dare reassure him that having a child with a disability wasn't the end of the world. At that point, six years into J.P.'s diagnosis, thirteen years into being his mother, and only a few years past the violent upheaval of his puberty, I did not know if I could promise that loving a disabled child was not the end of the world, at least the world as he knew it.

"Only connect," E. M. Forster famously said, and in that cab the scientist and the mother connected. That was the vision of two fragile X parents in Massachusetts who in 1994 decided to find a cure for fragile X and, along with a third parent, created the organization known as FRAXA, the Fragile X Research Foundation. Mike Tranfaglia and Katie Clapp, husband and wife, seek out and fund scientists who work on all fronts of the puzzle posed by this mutation. As of today, they have funded over eleven million dollars' worth of research.

One day in 1993 I received a phone call from Katie Clapp, who had somehow gotten my name as another parent of a child with fragile X. I was sitting in my kitchen in the house Harry and I had shared until the previous year, and feeling quite alone. Katie was vivacious and talked up a storm, and I liked her right away. Talking to another fragile X mom who wasn't my sister was too good to be true. We decided to meet for lunch the following week at a restaurant in between our houses, which were about an hour apart.

Over salads and iced tea Katie and I couldn't stop talking—about what it felt like to mother a child who had public meltdowns; about how our husbands handled it; about how our previously golden lives had changed. Katie and Mike had met as undergraduates at Harvard and had gone on together to the University of North Carolina at Chapel Hill, Katie for an MS in computer science and Mike for a medical degree. With all our education, the four of us had never imagined having children who would never go to college.

As Katie told me that day, she and Mike dreamed of finding a cure for fragile X through gene therapy. Since fragile X is a single-gene affliction caused by the lack of a single protein, they believed that a cure might be as little as five years away. Although, as the next few years would show, gene therapy turned out to be a lot more complicated than scientists had envisioned, that is still a distant goal of some FX research. The tantalizing knowledge that in fragile X, unlike some other disorders, only a single gene has gone awry, creates hope that someday a copy of that gene can be directly injected into the brain cells. This would be accomplished in a viral vector, a virus that has been stripped of its potential to harm and engineered to serve as a delivery vehicle for a gene. The challenge of gene therapy is always how to get the virus into the right cells in the body, not just the cells around the injection site. Then there is the need to express just the right amount of FMRP—not too much and not too little—to correct the deficits associated with the syndrome.

Gene therapy seems more distant now than it did when Katie and I first talked. So does the notion that we can reactivate the gene by reversing its methylation or chemical shutdown. It is common in the fragile X scientific community to speak of "flipping the switch" and "turning on" the FMR1 gene, but the mechanical simplicity of this metaphor belies the exquisite complexity of the body's genetic machine. Where biologists once believed that each gene makes only one protein, now we know that a gene codes for multiple proteins by splicing to alternate among them. That's why the human genome turns out to be much smaller than anyone expected: 30,000 genes can do the work that scientists once believed required 100,000. To complicate matters, recent research on fragile X has uncovered a couple of genes that are homologous with FMR1 but located on chromosomes 3 and 17 rather than the X chromosome. Dubbed FXR1 and FXR2, they encode proteins that are highly similar to FMRP. It seems the plot thickens every time a new clue appears in the lab.

Another hope is that the protein FMRP can be produced in drug form and injected like insulin for diabetics, keeping the synaptic connections well oiled and the cortisol squelched. However, FMRP plays a complex regulatory role, acting on other genes, on the neurons, and even on its own expression. It would not be a simple matter to control its expression in the human body.

For at least a decade researchers have known that the brains of patients with fragile X are abnormal, resembling immature, developing brains. The dendritic spines, structures on the neurons where the synapses form and signals are passed from one neuron to another, are long and thin rather than healthily stubby. Like a variation on the old joke that the food was not only awful, there wasn't enough of it, these fragile X dendritic spines are not only immature, they are overly abundant. You might think having lots of places where communication can take place is a good thing, but it's not, because it creates a kind of static. Healthy brains prune away excess spines to facilitate clear messages. Moreover, these skinny dendrites are not as efficient as their heftier normal cousins at creating contact between the cells.

The latest breakthroughs in curing fragile X involve basic research on protein synthesis at the level of dendrite and synapse, and promise to discover potential drug therapies to restore function at the synapses. In an exciting paper published in May 2002, researchers Mark Bear, Kimberly Huber, and Stephen Warren proposed a theory that the psychiatric and neurological aspects of fragile X—symptoms like anxiety, increased sensitivity to tactile stimuli, and seizures—are a consequence of exaggerated responses to the activation of a group of neural receptors called metabotropic glutamate receptors (dubbed mGluR's) that in turn affect protein synthesis. It appears once again that fragile X is really (if neurons are more real than the impulses they animate) a disease of excess, and the obsessions, hyperactivity, and sheer extravagance of my son's persona have their source in some over-excitable nerve endings in his brain. When J.P. freaks out at a fireworks display, his outburst is nothing compared to the explosions going on among his neurons. My ineffective pleas for him to calm down and take a deep breath may yield in the pharmacologic future to the dampening effects of an mGluR5 antagonist.

ON THE FIRST NIGHT of the National Fragile X Foundation conference in Asheville, participants were offered a tour of the nearby Biltmore estate, "America's largest home," followed by a reception and banquet. It was a stifling summer night, and the ornate wooden walls of this sixteenth-century-style French chateau seemed to weep with the southern humidity. Along with my sister Ann and her husband, James, who had also come to this conference, I moved languidly through a surreal opulence. Eventually I found myself, cocktail in hand, talking to a group of scientists from the Netherlands. One of them, I was excited to learn, was Dr. Ben Oostra, who, along with some other scientists, had created the first fragile X knockout mouse in his lab in the Netherlands, so called because the FMR1 gene is knocked out and a nonfunctioning copy inserted. These mice provide a vital model to study the FX mutation, even though it turns out that they are not quite as severely affected as their human counterparts. Something about a mouse seems to resist the full brunt of a life without FMRP. Nonetheless, these mutant rodents have enlarged testes, are hyperactive, and are not too swift in acquiring "novel spatial information" (translation: they can't find their way out of an unfamiliar maze).

I, of course, find them utterly charming. Jackson Laboratories, one of the sources of knockout mice, promises on their Web site that their JAX mice represent the "gold standard for genetic purity." A phrase that in other contexts would send chills down my spine here, among the experimental mice, lifts my heart. I look up the FMR1 knockout, the mutation made by Dr. Oostra—Strain B6.129P2-Fmr1$^{tm1Cgr/J}$—and see that it has macroorchidism, learning deficits, and hyperactivity (sounds familiar). When I click on the link marked "Diet Info," I half expect to see nachos, Sprite, and hamburgers instead of ground wheat, ground corn, fish meal, dehulled soybean meal, brewer's dried yeast, and lots more that J.P. would never eat. Two pairs of these genetically engineered mice cost $1,900, the price of cryorecovery from frozen mouse embryos.

When I imagine these knockout mice—represented on another company's Web site as cartoon mice in little boxing gloves—I can't help but see a tiny champion for my son and his cousins. I imagine these little guys failing to locate a hidden platform in a water maze, swimming slower than their normal littermates, paddling frantically with their tiny paws but never catching up. Little do they know they are doing just the right thing—failing to be normal in ways that might explain some of the things J.P. and his fragile X fellows do.

Ben Oostra and several colleagues tried to correct the effects of the fragile X mutation by introducing an intact copy of the FMR1 gene into the knockout mouse. "Rescue mice," they called the transgenic creatures they constructed, and they achieved success in ameliorating some aspects of the fragile X phenotype. Of course, the insertion of a gene into a human embryo raises ethical problems that are insoluble at this point, but other questions, too, haunt the promise of gene therapy to correct fragile X syndrome.

Can the future change the past? No one knows whether a person already living with fragile X syndrome can reap the benefits that theoretically would come from a working FMR1 gene. What would an infusion of FMRP mean to a person whose brain was formed dry of protein—someone like J.P.? In that desert for twenty years now, he has blinked his eyes at sunlight, his eyes have spun to whirl the world into focus, he has flapped his hands to locate himself in space, he has tingled at the slightest touch, he has felt the blood rush when he was forced to look into another's eyes. J.P.'s body took its shape in the off-kilter world of his mind: his calloused hands where he bit down to channel the surge of sensations, his flat feet with their shuffling gait, his head often turned askew to block your gaze. His brain bears the traces, there can be no doubt, its lanky dendrites hanging loosely like empty hands.

Who would J.P. be post-FMRP, in a life delivered de novo? ("I was yelling, 'Let me out! Let me out!'") Would he recognize the world in which he had grown up, now calibrated to just the right pitch for his comfort? Or would that world fail to hang together, like the nightmarish spectacle experienced by Oliver Sacks's blind man given sight, who did not find a paradisiacal normality in being able to see but a hellish denatured world that made no sense? Would the world recognize J.P.? Would I know my son? ("It's me, J.P.!") Would he know me? ("Now you're *who you are!*")

G. K. Chesterton coined an adage: "Do not free a camel of the burden of his hump; you may be freeing him from being a camel." Is J.P.'s essence the weighty burden of those extra CGG repeats? I honestly don't know, but I hope not. I imagine a J.P. who can read Walt Whitman with me, who can play softball with his father, who can jump in a car (my Honda? take it!) and drive off with a beautiful girl...marry her, have children—but I don't know this J.P. Would I like to know him? You bet I would, with every ounce of blood in me.

But I wouldn't give up the J.P. I have to know that other J.P. I wouldn't want to live without his wide-open love, his puckish humor, his extravagant Shakespearean language. Can I have those, too, I beg the engineers of the new and improved J.P.? Can I have my perfect boy along with the Perfect Boy? But they cannot answer me; they make no promises.

ONCE IN A WHILE the pain and the joy collide, and it's the sharpest way I know just who I am. It happens like this: I'm looking at a Christmas card sent by some friends from graduate school. Their three teenage children, bright-eyed and bursting with life, stand on a beach together, their arms linked. Most days I smile and toss these cards onto the stack, but today, for a moment, the tears well. I think back to the days when Harry and I imagined our children this way, when I didn't know a gene from a chromosome, when our biggest challenge was how to finish a research paper or the giant cocktails at Callahan's Restaurant.

But this is a split second of nostalgia, for J.P. and I no longer have time for the past. We are rushing on into the future, riding on the back of the rapid-fire gibbering of a mysterious code that stretches out, it seems at times, beyond the number of repeats inscribed on our genes, into the giddy unmapped regions of infinity.

J.P. asks, "And then what? And then what? And then what?" And somewhere down the echoing years, maybe I'll know the answer.

# Appendix

## *Resources for Fragile X Syndrome*

Fragile X Syndrome is one of the most common genetic diseases in human beings, occurring in all races and ethnic groups. Families like mine live all over the world—in Brazil, Italy, South Africa, India, China, the United Kingdom, Mexico, and more than a hundred other countries. Our children's skin and hair may be dark or light, but our kids flash the same shy smiles from faces subtly marked with the mutation they share. We spell *love* in many different languages, but always with an X.

The two organizations that I have found most helpful are the National Fragile X Foundation and FRAXA: The Fragile X Research Foundation. The mission of the **National Fragile X Foundation** is "to enrich lives through educational and emotional support, promote public and professional awareness, and advance research toward improved treatments and a cure for Fragile X." The foundation has a comprehensive Web site with information for parents, educators, and doctors, and is often the first place parents turn for help when their child is diagnosed. Every other year, the foundation holds an international conference that draws a unique mix of scientists, clinicians, educators and parents. The most recent conference, the organization's tenth, offered five days of more than a hundred sessions ranging from scientific presentations to hands-on calming therapy.

FRAXA was founded in 1994 by three parents of children with fragile X, Katie Clapp, Michael Tranfaglia, M.D., and Kathy May, to support scientific research aimed at finding a treatment and a cure for fragile X. FRAXA directly funds promising research, over eleven million dollars so far, and also provides support to families affected by fragile X and raises awareness of fragile X. My friends Mike and Katie have created a grassroots organization that proves that nothing succeeds like the passionate dedication of parents who want to give their children a better life.

The **FragileX Listserv** is a resource that didn't exist when my son was a baby. It would have been comforting to have been able to share problems and solutions with other parents around the world at any hour of the day or night. Located on a server at Emory University, it can be accessed via the "Get Involved" page on FRAXA's Web site.

Those seeking a book with practical information for parents should read the very useful *Children with Fragile X Syndrome: A Parents' Guide* (Woodbine House, 2000), edited by Jayne Dixon Weber.

Even today it can be difficult to find doctors and other medical clinicians who are knowledgeable about fragile X. When J.P. was diagnosed in 1993, the FX gene had been discovered only two years earlier, but today there are many more centers of expertise including a new clinic, funded by FRAXA, at **Children's Hospital Boston,** the very hospital that failed to diagnose J.P.

Dr. Randi Hagerman, the doctor who treated J.P. at the Fragile X Clinic at Children's Hospital in Denver, has since moved, along with many of her colleagues who specialize in fragile X, to the **M.I.N.D. Institute** at the University of California, Davis. However, some of the therapists and psychologists who used to work with Dr. Hagerman have stayed in Denver and founded **Developmental FX**, a center that provides therapeutic services for fragile X and other neurodevelopmental disorders. Another important center of treatment and research is the **Carolina Fragile X Project** at University of North Carolina, Chapel Hill.

For additional insight on therapies and educational options, parents can also look to organizations that serve children with conditions other than fragile X. The challenges facing those with fragile X are not unlike those associated with other developmental disabilities, particularly autism or pervasive developmental delay, as the story of J.P.'s many earlier diagnoses illustrates. Even though J.P. was not correctly diagnosed until age seven, he had already received the best interventions and education available because his therapists and teachers treated his symptoms and behaviors (attention deficit, delayed expressive language, low muscle tone, anxiety), some of which were shared by classmates with other diagnoses. In fact, J.P. has never gone to school with another person with fragile X, but he has had plenty in common with his classmates.

The overlap between fragile X and autism is the object of some intriguing current research, most notably a study funded by a partnership of nine organizations, including the National Institutes of Health and FRAXA, on the "Shared Neurobiology of Fragile X Syndrome and Autism." The NIH announcement of the study indicates that "between 2.5% and 6% of autistic individuals have FXS, and approximately 15% to 25% of children with FXS have autism. An additional 50% to 90% of children with FXS have some symptoms and associated features of autism, including poor eye contact, hand flapping, hand biting, speech perseveration and other language abnormalities, and tactile defensiveness." Scientists suspect there is "a common etiological or pathophysiological pathway between the two conditions" and are seeking to identify targets for new drugs they hope may treat both disorders. Details of the grant are on the NIH Web site; search for the Program Announcement number PA-05-108.

Along with all those who find themselves challenged by mutations on their genes or some other inscrutable biological destiny, J.P. and I will be watching and waiting in the years to come.

**National Fragile X Foundation**
www.nfxf.org
P.O. Box 190488
San Francisco, CA 94119
Phone: (925) 938-9300
Toll-free: (800) 688-8765
Fax: (925) 938-9315
E-mail: NATLFX@FragileX.org

**FRAXA—The Fragile X Research Foundation**
www.fraxa.org
FRAXA Research Foundation
45 Pleasant St.
Newburyport, MA 01950
Phone: (978) 462-1866
Fax: (978) 463-9985
E-mail: info@fraxa.org

**Conquer Fragile X**
www.conquerfragilex.org
P.O. Box 128
Palm Beach, FL 33480
Phone: (561) 833-3457
Fax: (561) 833-8791
E-mail: mail@cfxf.org

**Fragile X Research Foundation of Canada**
www.fragile-x.ca
167 Queen Street West
Brampton, Ontario
Canada L6Y 1M5
E-mail: fxrfc@on.aibn.com

**Fragile X Society (UK)**
www.fragilex.org.uk
Rood End House
6 Storford Road
Great Dunmow
Essex CM6 1DA
Phone: (44) (0) 1371-875100
Fax: (44) (0) 1371-859915
E-mail: info@fragilex.org.uk

# Acknowledgments

I remember where I was when I first realized there was poetry in all of this. It was June 1993 in Albuquerque, New Mexico, and I was listening to a speaker on the last day of the biennial conference of the National Fragile X Foundation. My son had only been diagnosed with fragile X eighteen months before, and every word I was hearing at the conference was like a punch to the gut. I sank down into my chair in the darkness of the auditorium as the implications of the diagnosis unfurled in slow motion before me.

Stephen Warren, professor of human genetics at Emory University Medical School and one of the leading researchers in the field of fragile X, was speaking on the molecular and clinical correlations of fragile X. He casually referred to the origin of the mutation as "a slippage in the primordial chromosome." Something about this phrase—the suggestiveness of the image, its elegant assonance, the conjuring of ancient ancestors—spoke to me. It reawakened another part of me that was not the devastated mother but the professional lover of literature, the student and teacher of poetry. The moment was just a tiny glimmer in the darkness of those days in New Mexico; I jotted down the words in my conference notebook and then lifted my head to listen to the bald facts of this new world. But I never forgot the phrase and I always knew that someday, when my feet were firmly on the ground again, I would return and explore what I might see by that glimmer of light.

And over a dozen years later, here I am.

I could not have written this book when I was younger. The demands of being the mother of a boy with fragile X, the disruption of divorce, the grieving that I had to do, my job—all these stood in the way. More crucially, perhaps, insight into what my life had become only evolved over time. I now have more perspective on the events of the past years, and have grown into my role as J.P.'s mother.

This book is as much my baby as the baby whose birth inspired it. As I began a leave of absence from my job as associate dean at Boston College to work on this book in earnest, I dreamed every night for the first ten days of a baby. Each night's baby was more adorable than the next. Finally one night the dream baby sucked a pacifier with a quivering chin, and I felt that, objectively and absolutely, this was the most adorable baby in the world. It was like a religious belief. When I awoke, I realized the baby in the dream was J.P.

I am grateful to Boston College, particularly to Joe Quinn, the dean of the College of Arts and Sciences, for allowing me to take a leave from my job to write this book. Thanks to Ourida Mostefai, who filled in for me during my leave, and the ongoing support of my assistant Carol Cianfrocca, my office was in better shape when I returned than when I left it. Of course, one needs a room of one's own, especially when the subject of one's book is laughing loudly at Oprah in the room next door, so I thank Boston College for providing extra office space and Wellesley College for lending me a space in the Clapp Library. I also enjoyed the use of my town's public library, the Wellesley Free Library, where J.P. works as a volunteer.

My writing group has provided me with constructive suggestions and warm support; I am so glad to know Steven Lee Beeber, Eileen Donovan-Kranz, Patrick Gabridge, Gregory Lewis, Diana Renn, Heather Holt Totty, and Deborah Vlock. I am especially grateful to Helen Vendler, who served as first reader on my dissertation many years ago in graduate school, for her continued friendship and keen advice. It was her fertile suggestion, over dinner at the Elephant Walk, to include poems in each chapter of the book. I will always appreciate Ben Birnbaum, editor of *Boston College Magazine,* for being the first to publish one of my essays. I owe a special debt to Michele Fishel for helping me find my voice and the courage to use it.

Richard Parks, my agent, took me on as a client even though I had never published a book. He has unfailingly treated me as if I were a bestselling author, and I owe him a lot. My editor at Beacon Press, Christine Cipriani, saw something in my book that she thought worth saying to the world, and I thank her for her meticulous attention to my manuscript.

Dr. Michael Tranfaglia, who, with his wife Katie Clapp, runs FRAXA, the Fragile X Research Foundation, generously explained to this scholar of literature the scientific theories behind current research into fragile X. I also want to thank Louise Staley-Gane for answering my questions on genetics. Any errors are very much my own. I would also like to thank the National Fragile X Foundation, which has invited me to speak at several of its biennial conferences. I thank Robert Miller, the foundation's executive director, and Deborah Kwan, its programs coordinator, for their encouragement and support.

This is a good place to thank all of J.P.'s teachers, therapists, doctors, and caregivers through the years. J.P. has opened up to me a world of people who understand and appreciate the uniqueness of every person. Some of you have been named in the book, as you are an integral part of our story. Others too numerous to mention have enriched our lives. J.P.'s parents could never have done it without you.

J.P. has a Y chromosome, too, and that comes from his father, Harry L. Manion III, who has passed on to J.P. his charisma and zest for life. Thanks, Harry, for your financial support, without which writing this book would have been even more challenging, and most of all, thank you for your never-flagging love for our son.

To my family, with whom I share this genetic heritage, with its harsh challenges and profound mysteries, I offer my book as a gift. Since the day I passed on the news that rocked our world, you have struggled along with me to carry this burden. I cannot put the troubles back in the box, but I can celebrate, quite simply, who we are. I thank my mother and father, Mari and Jack Dunsford; my sisters, Cathy, Maggi, and Ann; my brother, Mark; and my nieces and nephew for allowing me to tell our family's story and for supporting me in living it. And I thank those family members who died before the language of DNA became familiar to us: you also made me who I am.

To Stephen Pfohl, the man who barked back, my White Rabbit, your love and support sustains me every day. Thank you for giving me confidence when I felt I couldn't write a word, and thank you for sharing the Wonderland that is my life.

Finally, to John Patrick Manion, my son, my perfect boy—you have, literally, made me who I am today. And that's the biggest tribute of all.

# Credits

The names of some individuals and places discussed in this book have been changed to protect their privacy.

Chapter 5, "Base Pairs," originally appeared, in slightly different form, in *The Kenyon Review* (winter 2006) as part of the special section on the Human Genome Project, "Writing in Code."

Chapter 7, "Repeats," originally appeared, in slightly different form, in *X Stories: The Personal Side of fragile X syndrome*, eds. Charles W. Luckmann and Paul S. Piper (Bellingham, WA: Flying Trout Press, 2006), pp. 52–70.

Parts of Chapter 8, "Saltation: Coming Up for Air," originally appeared in *Boston College Magazine* (spring 1996) under the title "Heartstrings."

The quotations from *Alice in Wonderland* by Lewis Carroll in chapter 10 are from the Norton second edition, published in 1992.

The quotations from William Wordsworth's *Lyrical Ballads* in chapters 4 and 5 are from the Oxford University Press second edition, published in 1969.

"The Idiot," from *Complete Poems of Hart Crane* by Hart Crane, edited by Marc Simon, Copyright © 1933, 1958, 1966 by Liveright Publishing Corporation. Copyright © 1986 by Marc Simon. Used by permission of Liveright Publishing Corporation.

"The Motive for Metaphor," from *The Collected Poems of Wallace Stevens* by Wallace Stevens, copyright ©1954 by Wallace Stevens and renewed 1982 by Holly Stevens. Used by permission of Alfred A. Knopf, a division of Random House, Inc.